GOOD LIVING WITH Osteoarthritis

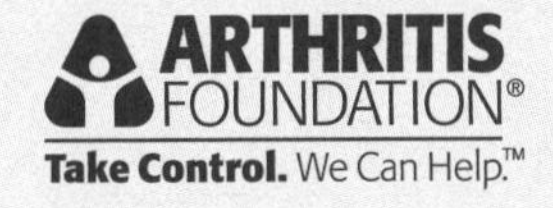

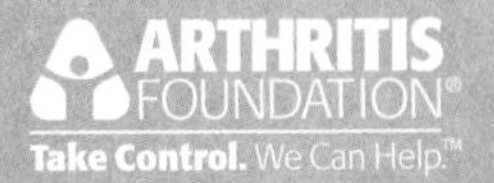

GOOD LIVING WITH
Osteoarthritis

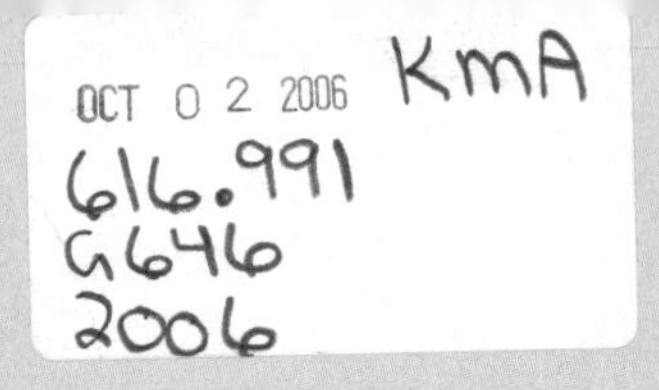

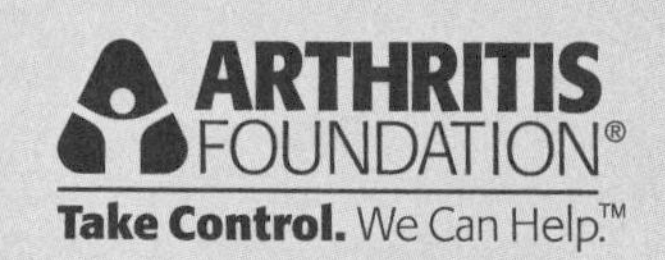

Printed in the United States of America
1st Printing 2000

This book is not intended as a substitute for the medical advice of physicians. The reader should regularly consult a physician in matters relating to his or her health and particularly in respect of any symptoms that may require diagnosis or medical attention.

Published by:
The Arthritis Foundation
1330 West Peachtree Street, NW, Suite 100
Atlanta, GA 30309

Library of Congress Card Catalog Number: 00-104036

ISBN: 0-912423-51-X

The Arthritis Foundation is proud to be a participating organization in the Bone and Joint Decade.

Participating Organization

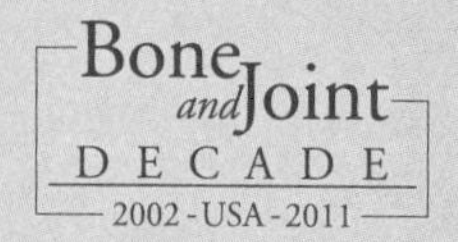

The mission of the Arthritis Foundation is to improve lives through leadership in the prevention, control and cure of arthritis and related diseases.

Table of Contents

FOREWORD

Osteoarthritis is, by far, the most common form of arthritis. Most recent estimates indicate that 21 million Americans – roughly 1 out of every 12 people – suffer from this form of arthritis. Osteoarthritis is associated with aging, so as the baby boomer generation gets older and people live longer, the number of people with this form of arthritis will increase substantially, especially over the next decade.

Differentiating osteoarthritis from the more than 100 disorders that affect joints presents little problem for doctors and requires little in the way of medical tests or procedures. Osteoarthritis targets key joints – most commonly those in the hips, knees, spine and ends of the fingers – each with characteristic signs and symptoms. For instance, people with osteoarthritis of the hip or knee generally note pain when getting out of a chair, climbing stairs or walking. Osteoarthritis is responsible for the vast majority of people who have chronic low back or neck pain. The condition also produces painful swelling of the finger joints that interferes with people's ability to do most things, including daily tasks like dressing and turning a key in a door, or pleasurable activities like sewing, playing the piano or holding a golf club.

A number of successful approaches are now available to prevent osteoarthritis, and to treat symptoms and improve joint function once the arthritis has begun. Regular exercise, weight control and avoiding injury to joints are critically important in both prevention and treatment, particularly for knee and hip osteoarthritis. Medications, including both over-the-counter and prescription drugs, play a very important role in pain management. Over the past decade, there has been a tremendous interest and increase in the use of alternative or complementary medicines for osteoarthritis, especially glucosamine and chondroitin sulfate. Finally, surgery to replace joints irreversibly damaged by osteoarthritis has become an almost routine procedure of immeasurable value to people immobilized as a result of hip or knee osteoarthritis.

The Arthritis Foundation believes that the actions people with arthritis choose to take play a large and important role in determining the outcome of their disease and the extent to which it impacts their lives. This is especially true for people with osteoarthritis. Education, self-help and taking personal responsibility are tools of empowerment and keys to achieving control of osteoarthritis. This book, *Good Living With Osteoarthritis*, is a practical and thorough discussion of osteoarthritis that will be of interest to the millions of people who suffer from the disease, and will hopefully guide them down a pathway to healthier lives.

John H. Klippel, MD
President and Chief Executive Officer
Arthritis Foundation, Atlanta, GA

ACKNOWLEDGMENTS

Good Living With Osteoarthritis is written for people who have osteoarthritis, as well as for their friends, family and loved ones. Bringing this book to completion was a team effort that includes the significant contributions of dedicated physicians, health-care professionals, Arthritis Foundation volunteers, writers, editors, designers and Arthritis Foundation staff.

Special acknowledgment should go to Shelly Morrow, who wrote the text. The chief medical reviewer of the book is John H. Klippel, MD, President and Chief Executive Officer of the Arthritis Foundation. The panel of medical reviewers of this book are David Felson, MD, MPH, Professor of Medicine and Epidemiology and Chief of the Clinical Epidemiology Unit at Boston University School of Medicine; Marc C. Hochberg, MD, MPH, Professor of Medicine, Division of Rheumatology and Clinical Immunology at the University of Maryland at Baltimore; and Leena Sharma, MD, Associate Professor of Medicine, Feinberg School of Medicine, Northwestern University.

Editorial director of this edition was Bethany Afshar. Art director of this book was Tracie Bullis. Dorothy Foltz-Gray edited this edition.

Introduction

INTRODUCTION
Your Role as a Self-Manager

When you're in pain and don't feel well, it can be easy to let other people make decisions for you. But you can learn how to take control of osteoarthritis yourself, playing an active role in managing your health.

This book will help you understand osteoarthritis and provide you with the tools you need to play a leading role in your own care. We'll look at how the disease may affect you, as well as successful ways to manage its symptoms.

What is a Self-Manager?

As you read this book, you'll see the term self-manager again and again. Self-managers are people who do just what's described above – they are informed patients who take control of their own situations.

A disease such as osteoarthritis can make you feel as if you're not in complete control of your life. You may not be able to do some activities as easily as you used to and you may need more help with certain tasks. But remember: You are in charge. Sometimes you will ask for help when you need it, and sometimes you'll find another way to get the job done.

Being a self-manager is an effective way to take – and keep – that sense of control over what happens to you. Basically, it means being informed about your disease and treatment options; following your treatment plan; communicating with your health-care providers; and managing your symptoms and the emotional aspects of your condition. The following overview will give you an idea of what self-management involves. These responsibilities are covered in depth later in the book.

The Five Habits of Successful Self-Managers

Now that you've read what a self-manager is, we'll look more closely at what successful self-managers do. The best way to become an effective self-manager is to study the following five habits and emulate them in your everyday life.

1. Learn as much as you can about osteoarthritis. (Chapters 1-2)

- Understand what osteoarthritis is and how it can affect your body.
- Keep informed by asking your health-care team questions and reading as much reliable

information as you can. Check your library or bookstore, and ask your health professional for other recommendations.

- Check with local hospitals, community centers and other health facilities to discover local resources such as classes and support groups.
- Contact your local chapter of the Arthritis Foundation (call 800-568-4045 or visit www.arthritis.org to find the office near you) for more information and resources.
- See the Resources section of this book for further information.

2. Join your health-care team. (Chapters 3-7)

- If you haven't done so already, see your doctor for an accurate diagnosis of osteoarthritis. Then, participate in planning your treatment program – and follow it. Your treatment may include medications, exercise, weight control and physical therapy.
- Write down questions and concerns to ask your doctor during your appointments.
- Keep track of your symptoms and mention any changes you notice to your doctor.

3. Develop a wellness lifestyle. (Chapters 8-10)

- In addition to following your treatment plan, follow healthy lifestyle habits, such as exercising regularly, getting enough sleep, maintaining your target weight and eating a healthy diet.
- Learn to manage stress effectively.
- Adopt a positive self-image and an upbeat attitude.

4. Assume responsibility for what you can control. (Chapters 11-12)

- Understand the difference between things you can control and things you can't. Then, take responsibility for what you can control.
- Learn to manage the physical aspects of osteoarthritis.
- Lose weight if necessary.
- Protect your joints.
- Accept what you can't control. Some symptoms won't go away.

5. Master emotional challenges. (Chapters 13-15)

- Find ways to manage emotional aspects of the disease, such as depression, stress and feelings of loss.
- Communicate openly and effectively with friends and family members about how osteoarthritis affects you.

The rest of this book is organized around these five habits, and we'll explore each one in detail to help you incorporate them into your life. We hope you'll find the habits useful tools as you learn to take control of your osteoarthritis.

PART ONE

Learn as Much as You Can

Chapter 1

Understanding Osteoarthritis: A Common, Chronic Disease

One of the best ways to become a successful self-manager is to learn as much as you can about osteoarthritis and its treatments. Knowledge is one of your strongest disease-management tools and the foundation of every other self-management habit in this book. Learning about the condition is an easy habit to start right away – and by picking up this book you're already on your way. In this chapter, we'll explain what osteoarthritis is and the process behind the disease. We'll also look at its history and causes.

What Is Osteoarthritis?

Osteoarthritis dates back to ancient times. In fact, recently discovered human skeletons from the Ice Age show signs of the disease. It's defined as a chronic condition in which tissue in the joint cavity known as *cartilage* breaks down. When this tissue deteriorates, bones rub against each other, causing pain and stiffness.

If you have osteoarthritis, you've probably heard this definition from your doctor. The disease may also be referred to as *osteoarthrosis, degenerative joint disease* or *degenerative arthritis.*

Chronic conditions like osteoarthritis last for several years or even a lifetime. The causes of osteoarthritis aren't yet known. Treatment may require a variety of medications and other measures, and these may change over time. Because this disease is long-lasting and can affect your day-to-day life for years, taking an active role in managing osteoarthritis is crucial. You can make a difference in how you feel by monitoring your symptoms, following your treatment plan and dealing with the daily challenges the condition brings.

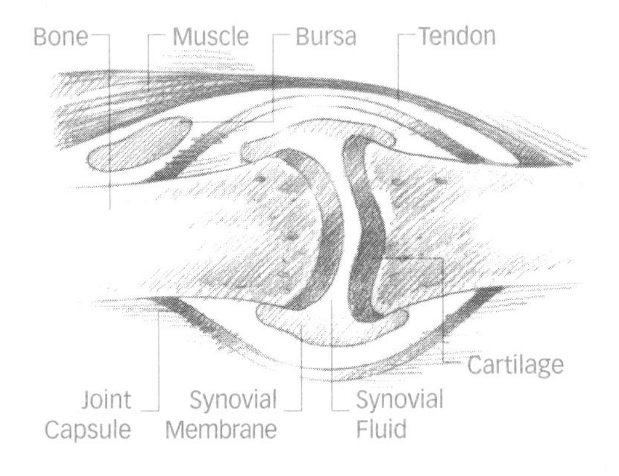

NORMAL JOINT

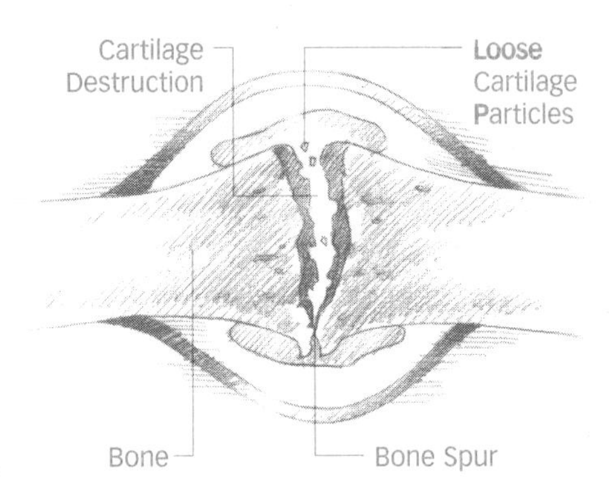

JOINT WITH OSTEOARTHRITIS

Unlike chronic conditions, acute ones such as a cold or the flu have a clear beginning and end, as well as a specific cause, such as a virus. They can be diagnosed with special tests, and many can be cured with drugs or medical procedures.

What Happens in Osteoarthritis?

When you have osteoarthritis, the cartilage begins to break down, usually gradually. As the cartilage wears away, the bones become exposed and rub against each other, a painful result. The deterioration of cartilage also affects the shape and makeup of the joint so that it no longer functions smoothly. You may notice a limp when you walk, or you may have trouble going up and down stairs because those movements put additional stress on the joint.

Other problems can occur inside the joint as cartilage breakdown affects the joint components. Fragments of bone or cartilage may float in the joint fluid, causing irritation and pain. Bony spurs, or *osteophytes*, can develop on the ends of the bones. Fluid inside the joint may not have enough of a substance called *hyaluronan*, which may affect the joint's ability to absorb shock. And although inflammation is not a main symptom of osteoarthritis, it can occur in the joint lining in response to the cartilage breakdown.

Who Gets Osteoarthritis?

If you have osteoarthritis, you're certainly not alone. Osteoarthritis affects approximately 21 million Americans, making osteoarthritis the most common form of the more than 100 arthritis-related conditions. In addition, osteoarthritis is one of the leading causes of arthritis-related disability in the United States. (Arthritis in general is the leading cause of disability among people age 15 and older.)

Osteoarthritis is common in people of all racial and ethnic backgrounds. Incidence of the disease increases with age, and it is most common in people over age 65. The disease occurs in men as well as women. Up to age 55, osteoarthritis is more common in men, but after age 55 it is more common in women. Women may be predisposed to osteoarthritis as they age, because their broader hips create an angle at the knees that makes them less able to withstand long-term stress.

What Causes Osteoarthritis?

Like other chronic conditions, osteoarthritis has no single, specific cause. Instead, there are several factors involved in the disease, including heredity and lifestyle. It may take a combination of these factors to cause osteoarthritis.

Osteoarthritis was once considered an inevitable part of aging. But researchers and doctors are learning more about how the disease develops and finding possible ways to control risk factors for osteoarthritis. By being aware of what puts you at risk for the disease, you can reduce the risk or minimize the disease's effects.

Factors Involved in Causing Osteoarthritis

- Heredity or genetic traits
- Obesity or excess weight
- Injury and overuse of joints

The Role of Genes

Scientists believe that heredity may play a role in osteoarthritis and are studying several genes that may be connected to the condition. The outcomes of these studies may help predict who is most likely to get the disease.

One possibility is that certain people may have a defect in the gene responsible for the body's production of collagen, the protein substance that makes up cartilage. This somewhat rare genetic defect might lead to abnormally weak cartilage that wears down after just a few decades of normal activity, causing osteoarthritis as early as age 20.

Other genetically based traits may result in slight defects in the way bones and joints fit together so that cartilage wears away faster than usual. The inherited trait known as joint laxity, or double-jointedness, in which the joints bend farther than the usual angles, may also increase the risk for osteoarthritis.

What Is a Joint?

Joints are some of the most ingenious structures in your body. They allow it to be flexible and to make almost any type of movement. But joints are subject to damage, especially when they are affected by osteoarthritis.

To understand arthritis, it helps to have a grasp of what joints are and how they work. Basically, joints are formed when two or more bones meet. You have different types of joints in your body that allow for different types of movement. Joints in the knees and fingers move like hinges. The ball-and-socket structure of shoulders and hips allows them to move in several directions. The facet joints in the spine allow it to flex, twist or rotate.

Soft-tissue structures around your joints can be affected by osteoarthritis. Muscles are made up of stretchable fibers that help move parts of your body. *Tendons* are fibers at the ends of muscles that connect them to bones. *Ligaments* are supporting tissues that connect bones at a joint.

Inside the joint, a strong, smooth tissue called cartilage covers the ends of bones. *Cartilage*, like ligaments and tendons, is primarily made of a protein called *collagen*. *Synovial fluid*, also called joint fluid, lubricates the joint to help it move smoothly. In osteoarthritis, the cartilage becomes rough and damaged, and tiny cartilage particles break loose in the joint fluid.

Just because you have inherited a gene that makes you more susceptible to the disease, however, doesn't mean you'll get it. In fact, researchers have found that some people who inherit the genetic risk for osteoarthritis don't wind up with the disease. So, a combination of factors may be required for the disease to develop.

The Impact of Excess Body Weight

Another factor that seems to influence osteoarthritis risk is excess body weight. You probably know that being overweight puts you at risk for heart disease and certain types of cancer, but it also can have a profound effect on your joints. The reason is that your major joints, such as knees and hips, already bear the brunt of your body's weight as you move through normal daily activities. Being overweight puts even more pressure on these joints.

For every pound of body weight you gain, your knees gain three pounds of added stress; for your hips, each additional pound translates into six times the pressure on these joints. After many years of carrying extra pounds, the cartilage that cushions your joints tends to break down more quickly than usual. Obesity may lead to osteoarthritis on its own, or it may combine with other factors such as your genetic susceptibility to produce the disease and worsen its symptoms.

Being overweight may be especially bad for your knees. Added pounds put a tremendous amount of stress on these joints each time you take a step. In fact, the strongest connection researchers have found between obesity and osteoarthritis is in the development of the disease in knee joints. Women who are overweight are especially at risk for damaging their knee joints.

Some research has shown a connection between being overweight and having an increased risk of osteoarthritis in the hands, but the reasons for that connection are unclear. But research has shown that weight gain, especially during middle age and later years, contributes most to an increased risk of osteoarthritis.

How Injury and Overuse Affect Joints

Sometimes repetitious movements or serious injuries to joints can lead to osteoarthritis years later. Some full-time athletes, for example, injure the same joints over and over, causing damage to the joints, tendons and ligaments that speeds cartilage breakdown.

Even joints such as shoulders, which don't bear much body weight and are unlikely to have osteoarthritis, can develop the disease after injuries or repeated stressful activities. For example, baseball pitchers who test the limits of their shoulder and elbow joints with numerous high-speed throws tend to develop osteoarthritis in those joints.

The constant knee bending required by some types of work, such as landscaping, can make cartilage wear away more quickly than moderate use of those joints. Osteoarthritis also tends to develop years later in joints where bones have been fractured or where surgery has been performed, such as in the knee.

Don't let these examples scare you away from exercise. Although overuse and injuries can contribute to osteoarthritis, the increased risk should not be viewed as a reason to avoid exercise. The risks of not exercising are greater than the risk of developing osteoarthritis from overuse. As you'll see later in this book, regular exercise can reduce the risk of osteoarthritis and help ease its symptoms. Plus, you can modify your activities to help minimize the potential risk.

Several other factors may contribute to osteoarthritis. These factors include other bone and joint disorders like *rheumatoid arthritis*; and certain metabolic disorders such as hemochromatosis, which causes the body to absorb too much iron; or acromegaly, which causes the body to make too much growth hormone.

What Is It Like To Have Osteoarthritis?

Now that you have a better understanding of what causes osteoarthritis and what it does inside your joints, let's look at symptoms you can expect to experience from the disease.

The first thing to remember is that the degree of pain or the specific joints involved may be different for each person who has osteoarthritis. Your knees may be affected so that walking is uncomfortable, while someone else may have painful fingers that make grasping and writing troublesome. Still, most people who have the disease have many common symptoms, including joint pain and stiffness, limited movement, and sometimes inflammation in the joint.

It is common for people with osteoarthritis to experience some stiffness in the affected joints after a period of rest, but that usually goes away after a few minutes of activity. You may find movement difficult at times, because you feel pain when you move or because your joints are stiff and require more effort to move. It also is common to experience joint stiffness in the morning, but this symptom usually lasts only for brief periods of 30 minutes or so.

Osteoarthritis occurs more often in certain joints. Generally, the disease affects joints that bear the majority of the body's weight, such as the lower back, hips, knees and feet. When these joints are affected, you may have difficulty with such activities as walking, climbing stairs and lifting objects.

Many people experience osteoarthritis in the neck and finger joints, including the thumb base. The elbows, shoulders and wrists usually are affected by osteoarthritis only when they have been overused or seriously injured. When finger or hand joints are affected, osteoarthritis can make it more difficult to grasp and hold objects, such as a pencil, or to do delicate tasks, such as needlework. Yet there are ways you can manage symptoms to keep the disease from affecting your life in these ways.

Can Osteoarthritis Be Prevented?

There are steps you can take to prevent osteoarthritis. In fact, osteoarthritis prevention really has two parts: preventing the disease in the first place and preventing disability once you have the disease. We'll begin by looking at ways you may prevent osteoarthritis from developing.

- **Be aware of family history.** Knowing your family history of osteoarthritis and other joint-related diseases is important. Although you can't do anything about the genes you inherit from your parents, you can find out if heredity puts you at increased risk. Did one of your parents develop osteoarthritis at a young age? Are you double-jointed? Do you have the wide hips, knock-knees or bow-legs that run in your family? By being aware that you may be predisposed to osteoarthritis, you can take steps that will reduce other risk factors and possibly stop the expression of those genes.
- **Control your weight.** As we've mentioned, being overweight is a significant risk factor for developing osteoarthritis. By maintaining a healthy body weight, you avoid putting additional stress on your joints. This stress can wear away cartilage more quickly than usual, and lead to osteoarthritis in weight-bearing joints such as the knees. Keep in mind that losing weight or avoiding weight gain from

What is Cartilage?

The main symptom in osteoarthritis is the breakdown of cartilage, which can lead to pain and limited motion in the joints. As we mentioned previously, cartilage is made mainly of a protein called collagen, which also gives skin its elasticity. Cartilage covers the ends of bones, and provides cushioning to prevent bones from rubbing together during movement and impact. It also offers a slick surface that allows your bones to glide against each other so your joints can move smoothly.

Healthy cartilage is strong and elastic. But when you have osteoarthritis, the cushioning cartilage surface wears away. As cartilage breaks down, bones rub together and joints no longer move as easily and comfortably as they did before. The result is the pain and stiffness of osteoarthritis.

Scientists once thought that damaged cartilage could not repair itself and regenerate like bones and other tissues can. Recent research has indicated, however, that in some cases cartilage can repair itself. Researchers are investigating this possibility, which may provide clues to better osteoarthritis treatments. Currently, experimental techniques to enhance cartilage repair have been successful only following an injury in people who have otherwise healthy cartilage. However, in the future such repair may be possible.

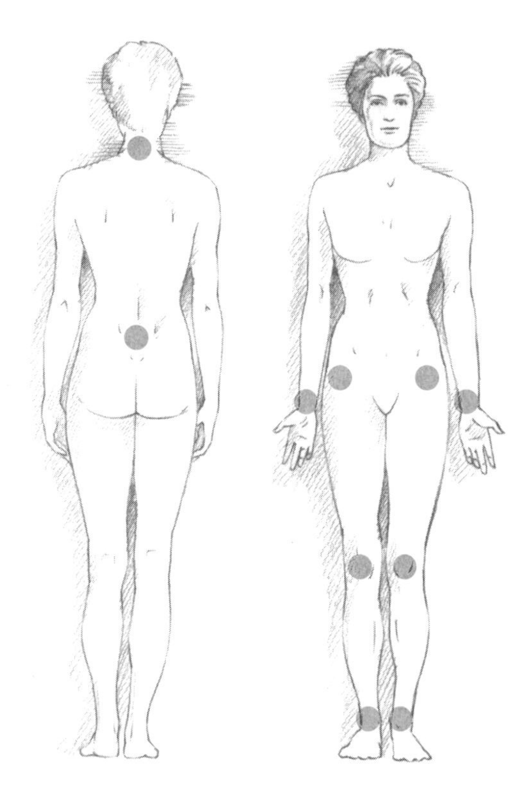

JOINTS USUALLY AFFECTED BY OSTEOARTHRITIS

middle age onward is the most effective way to avoid developing osteoarthritis or to lessen its symptoms.

- **Avoid damaging injuries.** Another important way to prevent osteoarthritis is to avoid serious injury to your joints. Injuries from routine falls or severe bangs and bumps during athletic activities can cause major damage to cartilage. These injuries can cause cartilage tears, or they can permanently alter the way your joints move so that they wear down cartilage more than usual. You can avoid injuries that may lead to osteoarthritis by taking care of your body. Warming up and stretching before athletic activity and exercise can help you prevent serious injury. If you do injure yourself, see your doctor to receive proper treatment. Injuries left untreated may heal improperly, which could lead to further damage later on.

Preventing Disability Once You Have Osteoarthritis

If you already have osteoarthritis, prevention is still a relevant issue. Although you obviously can't prevent the disease once you have it, you can prevent some of its effects on your body, and you can prevent structural progression and disability. These victories can be important, because they allow you to remain independent and do many of the activities you enjoy. You can protect your joints from further damage so that you maintain and even improve mobility in these joints. Listed at right are some ways to minimize the effects of osteoarthritis and protect your joints.

- **Maintain healthy body weight.** Maintaining a healthy body weight is an important way to ease pain in your joints and prevent further damage. Staying active and eating a healthy diet will not only make you feel strong and give you a radiant glow; it also will help you maintain – or reach – an appropriate weight. By not carrying additional pounds of body weight, you'll minimize the amount of stress placed on your joints. If you are overweight, losing just a few pounds can go a long way toward reducing your risk for osteoarthritis-related disability. Easing the pressure on your joints by shedding extra pounds can reduce pain in osteoarthritis-affected joints, which will help you feel and move much better. Later on in this book, we'll cover effective ways you can lose weight with simple exercise programs like walking.

- **Take frequent breaks.** Some jobs require repetitious motions – such as repeated knee bending to lift items in a warehouse or to stock shelves in a retail store – that can lead to joint damage over many years. If you have a job that requires doing the same motion over and over throughout the day, here are ways to reduce the effects on your body and help prevent further damage:
  - Even if you have only a couple of minutes to spare, walk around your workspace and stretch the muscles you've been using.
  - Exercise outside of work to help strengthen muscles so they can effectively support the joints you use during work.
  - Make sure that your work station is ergonomic, or properly designed and organized to support your body and reduce stress on it.
  - Use a comfortable chair with proper back support.
  - Position your computer monitor at eye level.
  - Take brief but periodic breaks, even if you remain at your desk, to stretch your back, neck and hands for relief. These breaks will help your body recover from the stress of repeated movement.
  - Use devices such as knee or wrist braces and splints to protect joints you have injured, especially when your job requires bending or heavy lifting.

As you can see, you can reduce your risks for developing osteoarthritis by taking good care of your body. If you already have osteoarthritis, you still can take steps to minimize the disease's effects. By following the advice given here, you can limit the impact of osteoarthritis, reduce pain and prevent future joint damage.

Chapter 2

Getting Informed:
Resources for Arthritis Education

Now that you understand what osteoarthritis is, you can learn more about it. An important part of learning about your disease is keeping up with the latest developments in research and treatment. New discoveries and treatment advances are occurring at an ever-increasing rate. And the wealth of health information available on the Internet has made medical research more accessible than ever.

Stay Up-To-Date

Keep abreast of developments in osteoarthritis research and treatment by paying attention to news reports about medical advances and by doing your own research. During appointments with your doctor, ask questions based on the relevant information you find.

Talking about new treatments can help you and your doctor evaluate your current treatment program and determine the appropriateness of any new options. The hype that surrounds new treatments may not always be backed by a great deal of reliable evidence. Reports or advertisements concerning new treatments can seem exciting at first; discussions with your doctor can help put the evidence in perspective and clarify the treatment's potential for you. For more information about assessing the validity of studies reported in the news, see "Evaluating News Reports about Arthritis" on page 15.

Resources for Information

A number of resources can provide more information about arthritis research or more in-depth coverage of advances. Here are a few of them, but keep your eyes open for other educational resources.

- **The library.** Your local library can be a great resource for magazine and newspaper articles that cover the latest research developments. You can search databases for recent articles on a particular topic. If you don't have a computer or Internet access at your home, most libraries now offer the use of the Internet for free.

If you're looking for studies published in medical journals, your community library may not carry these materials. Check with local university and medical school libraries instead.

If you have questions about searching the library's systems or the Internet, ask for help from the reference librarian. The library staff also can order books and other materials for you through Interlibrary Loan, a lending program established by the Library of Congress.

- **The Internet.** The Internet is a huge resource for up-to-the-minute health and medical information. But use your judgment: Anyone can put up a site and may not always post accurate and reliable information. Other sites may be designed to sell a product rather than provide unbiased information. Look for sites that are reputable, such as sites whose material is reviewed by physicians and medical professionals, or sites backed by health agencies like the National Institutes of Health or a university medical center. You also can search Medline, a service of the National Library of Medicine, for summaries of millions of articles from medical journals.
- **Organizations and agencies.** Many nonprofit health organizations and government agencies offer patient information on medical conditions. Often this

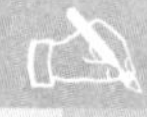

Personally Speaking STORIES FROM REAL PEOPLE

"I was diagnosed with juvenile rheumatoid arthritis at age 4. Since then, I have developed osteoarthritis as well. I am now 38 and married. We adopted our daughter from Korea when she was four months old. She is now 12 years old.

FOCUS ON THE POSITIVE

– RENEE LINDOW, IRON MOUNTAIN, MI

"I have had several surgeries due to the arthritis and have found that faith and the support of family and friends (the three F's) have been the most helpful to me in my daily life with 'Arthur.' Also, having a positive attitude is a must! I was taught from an early age to focus on what you can do, not on what you can't. My mottos are: 'Play the cards you are dealt' and 'F.R.O.G., Fully Rely on God.' I hope this helps someone."

Evaluating News Reports about Arthritis

When you hear medical news, you may have a hard time determining what a study's findings mean for you. It is tempting to believe results that point toward an end to your osteoarthritis pain. But be cautious in your assessment. The following guidelines will help you evaluate news about osteoarthritis.

- Does the information come from a respected publication or broadcast? Give more weight to reports that come from reputable media and medical journals.
- Did the study include a large number of subjects? Studies of just a few people tend to be less reliable than those with a large number of participants.
- Did the researchers study humans instead of animals? Research in animals is important, but the results aren't always relevant to people.
- Have the results been duplicated in another study? Results that occur in one study could be coincidental or the result of outside factors. Results that are repeated in several studies are more credible.
- Were the study participants evaluated over a long period of time? Studies that last a year or more usually provide more complete information.
- Did the researchers use a control group? Specific effects of a treatment are clearer when a study compares participants receiving the treatment to participants who aren't receiving that treatment. The control group may instead receive a placebo pill or procedure.
- Did the study follow one group of participants from start to finish using the same techniques? Studies that rely on physicians' past impressions or patient recollections tend to be less reliable.
- Does the study cite objective rather than subjective data? Results from patient reports or testimonials are less reliable.
- Is your doctor encouraged by the findings? If your physician doesn't think the report has merit, then it probably doesn't.

The more of these questions you answer with "Yes," the more likely it is that the study is reliable.

(Adapted from *Arthritis Today*. To order, call 800-283-7800 or visit www.arthritis.org.)

information is provided on the organization's Web site, but you can call or write to them to request it in the form of fact sheets, brochures and other written materials. These materials may be available free or for a small charge.

When you hear about some new treatment or other advance on the news, remember that organizations and agencies often draft statements about these reports. You can try looking for related position statements or press releases on the organization's Web site.

The Arthritis Foundation is one health agency that provides a wide selection of publications, books, exercise videos and other materials about arthritis. You can request free copies of brochures on such topics as osteoarthritis, exercise, managing pain, medications, surgery and more by calling 800-568-4045. Books on a number of arthritis-related topics are available at bookstores nationwide and by calling the Foundation at 800-283-7800. You can access the Arthritis Foundation and order products on the Internet at www.arthritis.org.

The Arthritis Foundation also publishes a bimonthly magazine called *Arthritis Today*, which covers the latest research, treatments and lifestyle management practices. You can find out about community resources, self-help programs, support groups, exercise classes and other activities through your local Arthritis Foundation office.

PART TWO

Join Your Health-Care Team

Chapter 3

Making the Diagnosis: Ways to Identify Your Disease

When you first experience joint pain and stiffness, you may not know exactly what the problem is. In fact, a number of conditions produce symptoms in the joints. Sports injuries, other types of arthritis and conditions that affect the soft tissues (such as bursitis or tendinitis) can cause joint pain and stiffness that may seem similar to osteoarthritis. To receive proper treatment, it's important that you see your doctor for an accurate diagnosis of your symptoms. A general rule of thumb is that if you experience joint pain for two weeks or more, you should see your doctor.

Seeing a Doctor

When people experience joint pain, most react by seeking a diagnosis from their primary care doctor. Even if your diagnosis is osteoarthritis, you may continue to receive most of your arthritis treatment from your primary-care doctor. Depending on the severity of osteoarthritis and how it affects you, you may also see an arthritis specialist (called a rheumatologist) for ongoing care or treatment.

Whatever the case, your primary-care doctor will probably remain involved in your arthritis care as a member of your health-care team. If you see a specialist, he or she will consult with your primary care doctor from time to time.

During your first appointment, your doctor will evaluate your symptoms and figure out what is likely to be causing them. He or she typically does this by taking a medical history, performing a physical examination and ordering some imaging or laboratory tests to confirm the diagnosis. The final diagnosis provides a basis on which you and your doctor can build an appropriate treatment plan.

What Is a Medical History?

Your medical history is information about your health background. It includes any diseases or conditions you have or have had; any allergies to medications or other substances; surgeries and medical procedures; and medical conditions that your parents, siblings and other close blood relatives have. Your doctor, a physician's assistant or a nurse will ask you some questions to find out this information.

The purpose of taking your medical history is to give your doctor important facts about your health history. Because certain conditions can be inherited, your doctor needs to know which ones run in your family. A previous medical problem could be influencing your health now. Having a record of your health background gives your doctor a better idea of what is going on inside your body.

While compiling your medical history, your doctor will also want to find out about the symptoms that prompted you to seek medical attention. By understanding what your doctor wants to know, you may feel more comfortable answering the questions, and you can provide the most accurate answers possible. Points your doctor may want to know include:

- a description of your symptoms
- details about when and how the pain or other symptoms began
- where you are feeling pain, stiffness or other symptoms
- how the symptoms are affecting you
- whether you have other medical problems that could be causing these symptoms
- whether your parents, siblings or other relatives have medical conditions such as arthritis that you may have inherited

As you answer the questions, don't feel that you have to be a medical expert or explain your answers in medical terms. Describing what you are feeling in your own words is most helpful to your doctor. If you have trouble, try thinking about your symptoms by using words that describe other familiar sensations, such as burning, grinding, sharp or achy. And think about the times when you notice the symptoms the most. Are they constantly with you, do they come and go, or do you have them for a few days and then they disappear for a while? Have they gotten better, worse or stayed the same over time or even during a single day?

Tell your doctor if your symptoms get better or worse at a certain time of day. Pain that increases during the day or becomes worse in the evening may indicate osteoarthritis. Your doctor can get an idea of what is going on by the way that you explain how you have been feeling. Point out, rather than describe, the areas on your body where you are experiencing the pain or stiffness.

Remembering what you want to tell your doctor when you're in his or her office can be difficult. The surroundings may distract you or make you nervous – and then after you've left, you think of something important you didn't mention. To make sure you don't forget, take some time before your appointment to consider what you want to say. The worksheet at the end of this chapter can help you make the most of your time at the doctor's office.

What's Involved in a Physical Exam?

A physical examination is another important part of making the diagnosis. During the exam, your doctor will look at your joints and touch those you've described as painful. He or she will be looking for areas that are tender, painful or swollen as well as indications that joints may be damaged. By touching your joints, your doctor can identify parts of the joint that seem enlarged, which could be the result of bony growths in and around the joint. Such growths are common in osteoarthritis. The doctor can see the pattern of joints that are affected, which helps determine the type of arthritis you are likely to have. For example, osteoarthritis typically affects the thumb base or the top two finger joints in an uneven pattern in the hands, but usually does not affect the wrists.

What Your Doctor May Ask You

Here are some questions your doctor may ask you during your appointment. Some are covered in the worksheet on page 28, which you can fill out before your visit.

- What is the main symptom or problem that made you seek medical attention?
- Have you been experiencing any other symptoms?
- How long have you had the symptoms? When and how did they begin?
- Do your symptoms affect your ability to work or perform other daily activities?
- Do you have any other medical conditions?
- Have your parents, siblings or other blood relatives been diagnosed with a form of arthritis?

To find out how arthritis is affecting your body, your doctor may ask you to stand up and move certain joints. This demonstration will show the range of motion in your joints, or how well you can move each joint through its full capabilities. In Chapter 9, we will discuss simple range-of-motion exercises you can perform at home. Joint disease such as osteoarthritis generally limits the amount of mobility you have in a joint and causes pain during movement. The doctor will observe you while you're standing to examine the position and alignment of your neck and spine. He or she may ask you to walk around the office a bit to see how you are able to move your hips and knees.

Joints Often Affected by Osteoarthritis

Osteoarthritis occurs more frequently in certain joints than in others. Examining which of your joints are affected helps your doctor determine if you may have osteoarthritis or some other joint condition. The following joints are those most commonly affected by osteoarthritis:

- Neck
- Lower back
- Base of the thumb
- Top two finger joints
- Knees
- Hips
- Base and joints of toes

What Tests Can I Expect?

The final part of making the diagnosis may involve laboratory tests to confirm the diagnosis your doctor suspects based on your medical history and physical exam. Blood tests usually are not helpful in diagnosing osteoarthritis because the disease does not greatly affect chemicals and special cells in the bloodstream that can be detected in these tests. Some of the most common tests used in diagnosing osteoarthritis are:

- **Joint aspiration** (or arthrocentesis). For this laboratory test, your doctor will administer a local anesthetic, then insert a needle into the joint in order to withdraw fluid. The fluid is then examined for evidence of crystals or joint deterioration. This test can help rule out other medical conditions or other forms of arthritis.
- **X-ray.** Imaging techniques like X-rays can show the physical effects of osteoarthritis to confirm the diagnosis. X-rays use radiation to penetrate the body's soft tissues and show internal structures like bones. The images can show damage and

Conditions That Can Look Like Osteoarthritis

Some symptoms of osteoarthritis can overlap with other conditions. Proper treatment of any condition depends on the correct diagnosis. If you haven't already seen your doctor about your symptoms, do so as soon as possible to get the care you need to feel better. The following conditions may have symptoms similar to those of osteoarthritis.

Rheumatoid arthritis. This disease causes joint pain and stiffness, but differs from osteoarthritis (see page 26). Rheumatoid arthritis involves inflammation of the joints, causing redness and swelling. Inflammation is not a major feature of osteoarthritis. Rheumatoid arthritis also can cause overall fatigue, fever and organ inflammation.

Polymyalgia rheumatica. This disease causes joint and muscle pain, as well as morning stiffness. It occurs mostly in people over age 50, which is an age when osteoarthritis symptoms often begin. However, polymyalgia rheumatica symptoms also include a general feeling of malaise and a high erythrocyte sedimentation rate, a measure of inflammation. Occasionally, polymyalgia rheumatica is accompanied by a fever.

Sports injuries. Sports-related injuries can occur in nearly any part of the joint or surrounding tissue, such as the muscle, ligament or tendon. They typically cause discomfort, pain and stiffness in the specific area soon after the athletic activity that caused the injury. Milder injuries tend to heal on their own within several days, but serious muscle and cartilage tears can require more substantial treatment, including surgery.

Bursitis and Tendinitis. These conditions involve inflammation of the bursae (small sacs found between bone and muscles, skin or tendons) or tendons (fibrous cords that attach muscles to bones). Because these conditions cause pain in the joint area and limit motion, they can be mistaken for arthritis. Bursitis and tendinitis, however, do not cause deformity, as arthritis can. Treatment usually includes rest and use of heat or cold to ease pain.

Fibromyalgia. This condition involves pain and stiffness in the muscles and tissues around the joints. People with fibromyalgia also experience increased sensitivity in certain areas of the body, fatigue and sleeplessness. They may feel at times as if they have a joint disease, but fibromyalgia, unlike arthritis, does not result in joint damage.

other changes in cartilage and bones that can occur with osteoarthritis.

- **MRI.** This acronym stands for magnetic resonance imaging. The MRI scanner creates a magnetic field around you as you lie on a table that slides inside a tunnel-like area. The waves produced by the machine form a picture of a specific area of your body. This test is more expensive than X-rays, but it does not involve the radiation risk of X-rays. And MRIs provide a two-dimensional view that offers better images of soft tissues such as cartilage to detect early abnormalities typical of osteoarthritis.

What's the Doctor Looking For?

By obtaining your medical history, doing a physical exam, and ordering appropriate tests, your doctor is looking for signs and symptoms that point to osteoarthritis. Unlike other diseases, osteoarthritis does not have specific findings that will show up in a lab test. Instead, the diagnosis of osteoarthritis involves a combination of the kinds of information mentioned in this chapter. Specifically, your doctor is looking for the following evidence:

- pain, stiffness and limited movement in the affected joints

Disease Differences

Osteoarthritis	Rheumatoid Arthritis
Usually begins after age 40	Usually begins between ages 15 and 50
Usually develops slowly, over many years	May develop suddenly, within weeks or months
Affects a few joints and may occur on both sides of the body; usually minimal; morning stiffness is common and may be severe but brief	Usually affects many joints, primarily the small joints on both sides of the body; prolonged morning stiffness of the joints
Affects only certain joints; rarely affects wrists, elbows or ankles	Affects many joints including wrists, elbows and shoulders
Doesn't cause a general feeling of sickness and fatigue	Often causes a general feeling of sickness and fatigue, as well as weight loss and fever

- bony enlargement of the affected joints
- X-rays that show formation of bone spurs
- X-rays that show a narrowing of the joint space from cartilage loss

What Your Doctor Should Tell You

There are a number of things you'll want to know once your doctor makes a diagnosis of osteoarthritis. This is basic information about your condition and its management, so be sure to ask your doctor if he or she doesn't explain the following:

- the results of your test and what these results indicate
- your treatment options and how they work
- when you should expect results from a prescribed treatment
- possible side effects of any medications and what to do if you experience side effects
- which changes in symptoms you should report to the doctor
- appropriate types of exercise and any lifestyle changes you should make
- resources for additional information
- when to make your next appointment and what to do between now and then

WORKSHEET: What to Tell Your Doctor

Writing down your concerns before your doctor's appointment and taking them with you ensures that everything you want to discuss gets covered. Think about these points before your appointment.

When the pain started ______________________________

____

What the pain feels like ______________________________

____

How long the pain usually lasts ______________________________

____

Time of day I feel the pain most ______________________________

____

Other symptoms I've noticed ______________________________

____

____

Other medical conditions I have ______________________________

____

____

Childhood illnesses I've had ______________________________

____

Adult illnesses I've had ______________________________

____

Surgeries I've had ______________________________

____

Medical conditions my family members have ______________________________

____

Chapter 4

Medical Managers: Working With Your Health-Care Team

As you manage your osteoarthritis, one of your most valuable relationships will be with your health-care team. Together, you'll monitor the progress of your disease and find the treatment plan that works best for you. In this chapter, you'll learn about all the medical professionals who may help you manage your disease.

Create a Successful Relationship

Finding the right doctor is key to creating a successful doctor/patient relationship. Discard the old idea of blindly following doctor's orders without discussion or question. You can – and should – take the lead role in your arthritis care. You'll need to find someone who not only meets high standards of medical knowledge and skill, but who also works well with your personality. Your relationship with your doctor should be a trusting partnership with open communication.

The doctor's philosophy of practice should mesh with your own expectations. Ask how involved patients are in decisions, the level of aggressiveness in treatment and the attitude toward prevention.

Members of Your Health-Care Team

For many people with osteoarthritis, the main medical professional they see is their primary-care doctor. Most likely, he or she will first diagnose your arthritis and will handle most of your care. If you are the general manager of the team, your primary-care doctor is the head coach. His coaching staff includes the nurses and other staff members in his office, who can answer some questions for you.

In some cases – when you need specialized medical care for a problem or complication, or for certain treatments – your primary-care doctor may refer you to another health professional. Your health-care team can include a number of health professionals with distinct areas of expertise. These professionals may be ongoing members of the team or periodic consultants for individual problems. Here's a brief explanation of what these professionals do and the roles they may play in your care.

- **Rheumatologist.** This type of physician is a specialist with advanced training in arthritis and related musculoskeletal conditions. Your primary-care doctor may consult a rheumatologist or refer you to one if he is uncertain what type of arthritis you have, or if he needs advice about a plan of treatment.
- **Osteopathic physician.** These doctors, also known as osteopaths or DOs (doctors of osteopathy) have the same level of training as medical doctors (MDs), but a different overall philosophy. Diagnosis and treatment stem from the idea that many illnesses are connected to disorders in the musculoskeletal system. These doctors tend to focus more on prevention and overall wellness than on the traditional medical model of treating disease. An osteopathic physician may be your primary-care doctor, or an osteopath may be a specialist, such as a rheumatologist.
- **Orthopaedic surgeon.** This doctor has specialized training in performing surgery on joints, bones, muscles and other parts of the musculoskeletal system. You may see an orthopaedic surgeon if your joints are damaged, and you need to consider a surgical procedure, such as joint replacement surgery.
- **Occupational therapist.** This health-care professional has training to help patients reach their highest level of independence in daily activities. An occupational therapist can teach you how to reduce strain on your joints during daily activities and can fit you with splints and other devices to reduce the stress on your joints.
- **Physical therapist.** This professional is trained and licensed in rehabilitation techniques. Physical therapists can help restore function and prevent disability for people affected by osteoarthritis. They can also design exercise programs to help reduce pain and improve the functioning of parts of your body affected by osteoarthritis.
- **Acupuncturist.** Acupuncturists are trained in the traditional Chinese medicine practice of acupuncture. The practice seeks to balance the body's vital energy, known as *qi* (pronounced "chee"), which is thought to be out of balance when you have a disease or illness. Acupuncture may help reduce pain for some people with osteoarthritis. See the section on acupuncture in Chapter 6.
- **Chiropractor.** Also known as doctors of chiropractic, these health professionals are trained in the practice of healing

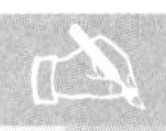

Personally Speaking STORIES FROM REAL PEOPLE

"For years after being released from the military, I continued to work. The misery of arthritis was always with me, but I never gave up – in part because of a positive aspect of my life called support groups. Never in my wildest dreams did I visualize myself in a support group. But I ended up in one. We have been meeting for the past six years once a month at our local library. And during that time, we've become a close group, almost like brothers and sisters.

MONTHLY DOSES OF HAPPINESS: SUPPORT GROUPS

– JOE DEMERS, MIDDLEBURG, FL

"Explaining what we acquire in these meetings is simple. Our camaraderie gives us that much needed lift, and we feel good after each meeting – so good that we stay together for lunch at one of the local eateries. Our meetings consist of much talking, getting things off our chests, some guest speakers, and most of all, being able to relate to others who understand what we are going through without any of those suspicious looks from the 'I don't see anything wrong with you' types. We do not feel sorry for each other. We don't allow it. But to be able to fill that terrible void by communicating with others who understand how we feel is truly a godsend.

"Now, I'm off to our support group for that monthly dose of happiness. For those who are skeptical, what do you have to lose? All you need to do is gather the right positive-thinking types and go at it. Feel free to ask the complainers to leave. Happy grouping."

through spinal manipulation. They may be helpful in treating certain back and neck problems, but they are not licensed to perform surgery or prescribe drugs. For more information, see the section on chiropractic in Chapter 6.

- **Registered nurse.** Nurses have professional medical training to carry out routine care under the supervision of a doctor. A nurse is likely to give you patient education materials and help explain how to follow the treatment plan your doctor prescribes. You may receive some of your care from a *nurse practitioner*, a registered nurse with additional training in medical therapies and treatments.
- **Podiatrist.** These doctors have special training in diagnosing and treating foot

problems such as bunions and hammer toes. If osteoarthritis severely affects your feet, you may see a podiatrist to help correct deformity and ease pain.

- **Pharmacist.** This health professional is licensed to dispense medicines. A pharmacist fills your prescriptions and can explain the drugs' actions and side effects. Pharmacists can answer your questions about prescription and over-the-counter medications.
- **Social worker.** A social worker is licensed to help people deal with the impact of chronic illness on their lives. Usually this involves helping people connect with social services and other types of assistance. Social workers can also help you with solutions to social and financial problems related to your disease.
- **Psychologist.** This health professional has specialized training in mental processes, especially as they relate to human behavior. A psychologist may provide counseling for people with osteoarthritis who need help in dealing with the emotional aspects of having a chronic illness.
- **Physiatrist.** A physiatrist is a physician who has additional specialized training in physical medicine and rehabilitation. This type of doctor may oversee your physical therapy program.

How to Work Together

Having a chronic illness like osteoarthritis requires that you monitor your disease through ongoing medical appointments. You'll be working closely with your health-care team to manage the condition. Establishing effective working relationships with the members of your health-care team is essential to taking control of your osteoarthritis and getting the proper treatment. As in any other relationship, the foundation of a solid partnership with your health-care team is good communication.

Like any patient, you want your doctor to tell you what is going on in your body. The reverse also is true: Your doctor wants to hear about changes in symptoms or remedies you try. You each have vital information about your condition that the other needs to know in order to fulfill your part of the treatment bargain.

One of the best ways to enhance communication with your doctor is by preparing for your appointments. Knowing what you want to tell your doctor and what questions you have can help you make the most of your time together during the appointment.

Use the following tips to keep good communication flowing between you and your doctor.

- **Share information.** Look at your appointments as opportunities to update each other on your situation. Tell your doctor about any changes in your symptoms and how you've been doing in following your treatment plan. Discuss anything that may not be working for you; self-care practices, such as exercise, that you've been following; and any complementary therapies you've tried. Some supplements, herbs, and over-the-counter medications could interact with your prescribed medications, so be sure to keep your doctor informed. Changes in your condition that may seem small could give your doctor additional clues about your disease, so don't keep changes to yourself.
- **Ask questions.** The Latin word for doctor also means "teacher," and education is part of your doctor's job. Your physician wants you to understand how to take care of yourself. If you don't understand what your symptoms mean, or part of your treatment plan such as how to take your medication, ask questions until you do understand.

Doctors are busy, and they may not have as much time to talk and answer questions as you may need during an office visit. If you're feeling rushed during an appointment, ask to schedule another time to talk so your doctor can answer your questions. Or ask if another qualified member of the staff, such as a nurse, could help you. Often, a nurse will have more time than the doctor to explain information about your treatment and medications. In fact, an important part of a nurse's job is to educate patients.

- **Monitor symptoms.** You may not always remember changes you've noticed or questions that have come up between doctor visits. You may find it helpful to

Initials You Should Know

Here's a brief rundown of some initials you may see next to a health professional's name and what these initials mean. The roles of these professionals are explained in this chapter.

DO: Osteopathic physician

MD: Medical doctor

PT: Physical therapist

OT: Occupational therapist

DC: Doctor of chiropractic

AAMA: American Association of Medical Acupuncturists

CA: Certified acupuncturist

RN: Registered nurse

DPM: Doctor of podiatric medicine

keep an informal journal or logbook of your symptoms and questions for your doctor. This exercise can help you recognize patterns in how you feel. And it may help you remember issues – how a certain medication is working, for example – that you want to share with your doctor. Before appointments with your doctor, review your log and questions. Put the most relevant issues on your list of things to discuss.

- **Listen.** Just as you want your doctor to be attentive to your concerns, you should listen carefully when your doctor is explaining something. A chronic illness requires you to do several new things, such as taking medications and doing helpful exercises, so there may be a lot to remember at first. You may want to use your journal to take notes on instructions and other important information.
- **Bring someone with you.** Consider bringing your spouse, a close friend or family member to your appointment. That person can provide support if you're feeling uneasy and can help you remember your concerns and your doctor's instructions.
- **Take time to review.** Before you leave each appointment with your doctor or other health-care provider, take a few moments to go over the main points you've discussed. Briefly review the answers to your questions, your health status and any new things your doctor has asked you to do. Make sure you've taken care of any prescriptions that need refills, and that you understand how to take any new medications.

Chapter 5

Medical Options: Drug Therapies for Osteoarthritis

Treatment is one aspect of managing your condition that you can take control of – first by taking part in devising your treatment plan with your health-care team and then by carefully following the plan. Understanding the available options will help you have productive discussions with your doctor and make informed decisions about your care. In the next two chapters, we'll cover the most common treatments for osteoarthritis, how they work and how they may help you.

Osteoarthritis can affect your body in a number of ways, from pain and stiffness in your joints to difficulty moving and performing everyday activities. And it affects your life in practical and emotional ways.

Because having a chronic illness like osteoarthritis touches nearly every aspect of your life, your management plan must do the same. An effective plan addresses you as a complete person, so it must cover strategies for your mind, as well as for your body. Osteoarthritis treatment should help your joints feel better, make your whole body feel well, and keep your mind healthy.

Methods include exercise and physical therapy, general health practices, medication, stress management and positive emotional responses. We'll look at ways to address all of these parts of osteoarthritis treatment in the next few chapters.

What Are the Treatments for Osteoarthritis?

It is important to understand that no cure for osteoarthritis exists right now. But by following the treatments and other strategies described in this book, you can lessen the disease's impact on your body and your life. Proper treatment includes a combination of therapies to control pain and other symptoms, improve your ability to function in daily activities and slow the disease's progress. Most treatment plans include some combination of the following elements:

- aerobic exercise
- weight control
- joint protection
- physical and occupational therapy
- medications

In severe cases of osteoarthritis, when the therapies listed above don't help, surgery may be considered. We'll discuss that option in more detail in Chapter 7.

Medications for Treating Osteoarthritis

Most people with osteoarthritis take some type of medication to ease the symptoms of the disease. Medications used to control osteoarthritis usually focus on relieving pain, but some newer medicines are targeting other symptoms and disease progression. Your doctor will work with you to find the drug or combination of drugs that works best for you.

Analgesics

Analgesics are drugs that relieve pain. These medicines do not relieve inflammation or swelling. But if pain relief is your main concern, these drugs tend to have fewer side effects than drugs that relieve inflammation.

The most commonly used analgesic is acetaminophen, which the American College of Rheumatology recommends for the treatment of mild-to-moderate pain caused by osteoarthritis. Acetaminophen is available over the counter as generic and store brands or as the name brands *Tylenol*, *Anacin* (aspirin-free), *Excedrin* caplets and *Panadol*. Acetaminophen can be taken in doses of 325 to 1,000 mg every four to six hours, but no more than 4,000 mg should be taken per day. This drug can cause problems if used with alcohol. Check with your doctor before using acetaminophen if you consume more than three alcoholic drinks per day.

If you have severe pain, your doctor may prescribe a stronger analgesic. Examples include propoxyphene hydrochloride (*Darvon*, *PC-Cap* and *Wygesic*), acetaminophen with codeine, and tramadol (*Ultram*). Often, these drugs are used only for short periods because they carry the risk of dependence.

TOPICAL ANALGESICS

These medications include creams or rubs that are applied directly to the painful area. These over-the-counter products are helpful if you have only a few affected joints or if oral medications alone aren't adequate. The most common active ingredients are counterirritants, salicylates and capsaicin. Never use topical products with heat treatments, because the combination can cause serious burns.

- **Counterirritants** include such substances as wintergreen oil, camphor and eucalyptus oil. They stimulate nerve endings, distracting the brain's attention from joint pain. Some product examples are *ArthriCare*, *Icy Hot* and *Therapeutic Mineral Ice*.
- **Salicylates** work in a similar way to an ingredient that is found in some oral

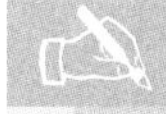

Personally Speaking STORIES FROM REAL PEOPLE

"Several years ago, I was diagnosed with osteoarthritis. In addition, I have lupus, a vascular necrosis and psoriatic arthritis, along with many other medical problems. And I am allergic to most of the drugs normally used to help pain.

"What has kept me going is a positive attitude and a philosophy to accept what you cannot control and do the best you can under difficult circumstances. I realize that most people are not really interested in my problems, and long ago, I learned that if I wanted to find sympathy, I'd have to look under 'S' in the dictionary. So, I try not to let people know what I am feeling and try to hide the pain as much as possible.

KEEP YOUR HANDS MOVING

– DORIS WIND,
KEW GARDEN HILLS, NY

"To be active is very important. I work full time in a very stressful environment, which puts great strain on me and often leads to flares. Doing lupus peer counseling on the telephone not only helps me but gives me a good feeling of helping others. It helps me realize that my problems are small, compared with the next person's problems.

"Hobbies that provide diversion and help me physically include knitting, needlepoint, embroidery and counted cross-stitch. I enjoy donating some of my knitting (sweaters, scarves and hats for teddy bears) to children in hospitals. Keeping my hands moving is important even though they hurt. I derive pleasure from giving to others.

"My children have been a big help with my arthritis. They realize what I am going through, and they do as much as possible for me. But I try to be as independent as possible because I don't want to burden them. Now, with great anticipation, I am looking forward to the birth of my first grandchild."

medications. They hamper the activity of prostaglandins, which are chemicals in the body involved in pain and inflammation. If you are allergic to aspirin, check with your doctor before using topical salicylate products. Some brand-name examples are *BenGay*, *Aspercreme*, *Flexall* and *Sportscreme*.

- **Capsaicin** is a natural ingredient found in cayenne peppers. It helps relieve pain by depleting a neurotransmitter that sends pain messages to the brain. Capsaicin products usually take a few weeks to work and can cause stinging sensations at first. Creams containing capsaicin are recommended by the American College of Rheumatology for treating knee osteoarthritis. You should not use the creams on broken skin or in conjunction with heat treatments, because a combination could cause serious burns. Take care not to let capsaicin products come in contact with your eyes. Examples include *Zostrix*, *Zostrix HP* and *Capzasin-P*.

Risk Factors for Ulcers or Stomach Problems

Stomach complications associated with certain medications can occur without warning, even in people who have never had stomach pain or heartburn. You may have a higher risk of stomach complications if one or more of the following risk factors are true for you. You may be at risk if you:

- Are over age 60
- Have severe disability from arthritis
- Smoke
- Have a history of ulcers or gastrointestinal bleeding
- Have a history of cardiovascular disease
- Consume more than three alcoholic drinks per day
- Use blood-thinning medications, such as warfarin
- Use cortisone medications, such as prednisone
- Are generally in poor health
- Have a *Helicobacter pylori* (*H. pylori*) infection

NSAIDs

Nonsteroidal anti-inflammatory drugs, or NSAIDs, are a large group of medications used to help reduce joint pain, swelling and inflammation. NSAIDs are available over the counter and by prescription. For patients with knee osteoarthritis who experience severe-to-moderate pain and signs of inflammation, the ACR recommends NSAIDs as an alternate initial therapy to acetaminophen. Aspirin (*Anacin, Ascriptin, Bayer, Bufferin, Excedrin* tablets) is the most common NSAID. Other examples of NSAIDs include ibuprofen (*Advil, Motrin IB, Nuprin*), ketoprofen (*Actron, Orudis KT, Oruvail*), naproxen (*Naprosyn, Naprelan*), and naproxen sodium (*Anaprox, Aleve*). Meloxicam (*Mobic*) is an NSAID available by prescription only.

NSAIDs work by stopping the production of chemicals called prostaglandins that occur naturally in the body and are involved in inflammation.

An important side effect to consider with NSAIDs is stomach upset and irritation, which can lead to stomach bleeding and ulcers (see the box on opposite page). To guard against this problem, your doctor may recommend taking these drugs with food or taking a stomach-protecting drug with them. The stomach irritation associated with NSAIDs can be increased by alcohol consumption, so check with your doctor before using these drugs if you consume more than three alcoholic drinks per day.

If you are allergic to aspirin, check with your doctor before taking any NSAIDs.

COX-2 INHIBITORS

COX-2 inhibitors (short for cyclooxygenase-2 specific inhibitors) are a third generation of more targeted NSAIDs. Research has shown that there are two types of enzymes involved in prostaglandin production. One type, known as COX-1, produces prostaglandins that help protect the digestive system from its own corrosive acid. The other type, called COX-2, is involved in the production of prostaglandins that play a role in inflammation.

Traditional NSAIDs inhibit both COX-1 and COX-2, which decreases inflammation but can cause damage to the stomach. Instead of affecting all prostaglandins, COX-2 drugs only stop production of erostaglandins, the type of prostaglandin involved in inflammation, without affecting those that protect the stomach (controlled by COX-1).

In theory, because they don't affect the stomach-protecting prostaglandins, the COX-2 drugs should be safer for the stomach than typical NSAIDs. However, they carry a risk of heart attack, stroke, blood clot or severe skin reactions. As of press time, celecoxib (*Celebrex*) is the only COX-2 on the market. Two other COX-2s were voluntarily pulled from the market because of the risks. Always talk to your doctor for the latest information on COX-2s.

Injectable Corticosteroids

Corticosteroids are drugs related to the naturally occurring hormone in your body called cortisone. In some cases your doctor may inject these drugs into a painful joint for fast, targeted relief. When fluid build-up in knee osteoarthritis, the doctor may drain fluid from the knee and then inject a corticosteroid medication. The American College of Rheumatology recommends corticosteroid injections as an alternate initial therapy for patients with moderate-to-severe knee pain and signs of inflammation who do not get relief from acetaminophen. You can have corticosteroid injections in the same joint only three to four times per year.

Hyaluronic Acid Therapy

One treatment specifically for knee osteoarthritis is *hyaluronic acid therapy,* also called *viscosupplementation.* Hyaluronic acid, a substance naturally found in joint fluid that acts as a shock absorber and lubricant, allowing joints to move smoothly over each other. However, the acid appears to break down in people with osteoarthritis. By injecting it in the joint it may lessen pain and inflammation. The injections are given once a week for three or five weeks, depending on the product (examples are *Synvisc* and *Hyalgan*). A small amount of joint fluid is removed first to make room for injecting the hyaluronic acid.

According to ACR guidelines, hyaluronic acid therapy may be helpful to patients who have had inadequate response to NSAIDs or COX-2 drugs, or who have experienced adverse side effects from these drugs. Clinical trials have shown that the injections may provide pain relief for people with mild to moderate osteoarthritis of the knee. Relief can last for several months. It is not yet known whether the injections are helpful for other joints. Side effects include reactions at the injection site. Hyaluronic acid products became available in 1998, and there is not yet a great deal of information available on the products' long-term effectiveness.

Because of the makeup of these products, most hyaluronic acid injections are not recommended for people allergic to bird feathers, bird proteins or eggs.

Drugs Used in Treating Osteoarthritis

TRADITIONAL NSAIDs: Nonsteroidal Anti-Inflammatory Drugs

With twenty prescription medications in the group – three of which are available in lower-strength, non-prescription doses – traditional NSAIDs are the largest subset of the NSAID class. Like all medications, NSAIDs, even non-prescription versions, carry a risk of side effects, including abdominal or stomach cramps, pain or discomfort; diarrhea; dizziness; drowsiness; edema (swelling of the feet); gastrointestinal bleeding; headache; heartburn or indigestion; nausea or vomiting; peptic ulcer. All NSAIDS may cause an increased risk of serious blood clots, heart attacks and stroke, which can be fatal. This risk may increase with dose and duration of use. Patients with cardiovascular disease or risk factors for cardiovascular disease may be at greater risk. These drugs should not be used for pain in people having coronary bypass surgery. For that reason, consult your doctor before taking any medication you buy without a prescription.

Do not take traditional NSAIDs with other prescription or OTC NSAIDS. Take as directed at the same time every day – and taken with food or an antacid. Do not take OTC NSAIDs for more than 10 days for pain or three days for fever unless directed to do so by a doctor.

Diclofenac potassium

Brand name: *Cataflam*
Dosage: 100 to 200 mg per day in 2 or 4 doses

Diclofenac sodium

Brand name: *Voltaren, Voltaren XR*
Dosage: 100 to 200 mg of *Voltaren* per day in 2 or 4 doses; or 100 mg of *Voltaren XR* per day in a single dose

Diclofenac sodium with misoprostol

Brand name: *Arthrotec*
Dosage:: 150-200 mg per day in 2 to 4 doses
Compared to other NSAIDS, this drug carries less risk of gastric ulcers but an increased one for abdominal pain and diarrhea.

Diflunisal

Brand name: *Dolobid*
Dosage: 500 to 1,500 mg per day in 2 doses

Etodolac

Brand names: *Lodine, Lodine XL*
Dosage: 600 to 1,200 mg per day in 2 to 3 doses for *Lodine*; 600 mg per day in a single dose for *Lodine XL*

Drugs Used in Treating Osteoarthritis (cont.)

Fenoprofen calcium
Brand name: *Nalfon*
Dosage: 900 to 2,400 per day in 3 or 4 doses; never more than 3,200 mg per day

Flurbiprofen
Brand name: *Ansaid*
Dosage: 200 to 300 mg per day in 2 to 4 doses

Ibuprofen
Prescription: *Motrin*
Non-prescription: *Advil, Motrin IB, Nuprin*
Dosage: 1,200 to 3,200 mg per day in 3 or 4 doses for prescription-strength *Motrin*; 200 to 400 mg every 4 to 6 hours as needed, not exceeding 1,200 mg per day, for the over-the-counter brands

Indomethacin
Brand name: *Indocin, Indocin SR*
Dosage: 50 to 200 mg per day in 2 to 4 doses for *Indocin*; 75 mg per day in 1 dose or 150 mg per day in 2 doses for *Indocin SR*

Ketoprofen
Prescription: *Orudis, Oruvail*
Non-prescription: *Actron, Orudis KT*
Dosage: 200 to 225 mg per day in 3 or 4 doses for *Orudis*; 150-200 mg per day in a single dose for *Oruvail*; 12.5 mg every 4 to 6 hours as needed for *Actron* and *Orudis KT*

Meclofenamate sodium
Brand name: *Meclomen*
Dosage: 200 to 400 mg per day in 4 doses

Mefenamic acid
Brand name: *Ponstel*
Dosage: 500 mg initial dose, then 250 mg every 6 hours as needed, for up to 7 days

Meloxicam
Brand name: *Mobic*
Dosage: 7.5 to 15 mg per day in a single dose

Nabumetone
Brand name: *Relafen*
Dosage: 1,000 mg per day in 1 or 2 doses; 2,000 mg per day in 2 doses

Naproxen

Brand names: *Naprosyn, Naprelan*
Dosage: 500 to 1,500 mg per day in 2 doses for *Naprosyn*; 750 or 1,000 mg per day in a single dose for *Naprelan*

Naproxen sodium

Prescription: *Anaprox*
Non-prescription: *Aleve*
Dosage: 550 to 1,650 mg per day in 2 doses for *Anaprox*; 220 mg every 8 to 12 hours as needed for *Aleve*

Oxaprozin

Brand name: *Daypro*
Dosage: 1,200 mg or 1,800 mg per day in a single dose

Piroxicam

Brand name: *Feldene*
Dosage: 20 mg per day in 1 or 2 doses

Sulindac

Brand name: *Clinoril*
Dosage: 300 to 400 mg per day in 2 doses

Tolmetin sodium

Brand name: *Tolectin*
Dosage: 1,200 to 1,800 mg per day in 3 doses

SALICYLATES

A subset of NSAIDs, salicylates work much like other NSAIDs to relieve pain and inflammation. Aspirin is the most familiar salicylate. In addition to side effects similar to those of other NSAIDs, frequent large doses of acetylated salicylates like aspirin may cause the additional side effects of confusion, deafness, dizziness, ringing in the ears, kidney problems, and gastrointestinal bleeding.

Chemical variations called *nonacetylated salicylates*, however, are associated with less stomach irritation, and they don't interfere with kidney function or blood clotting. But they also lack aspirin's protection against heart attacks and strokes.

ACETYLATED SALICYLATES

Aspirin

Brand names: *Anacin, Ascriptin, Bayer, Bufferin, Ecotrin, Excedrin tablets*
Dosage: 2,400 to 5,400 mg per day in several doses

Drugs Used in Treating Osteoarthritis (cont.)

NON-ACETYLATED SALICYLATES

Choline and magnesium salicylates
Brand names: *CMT, Tricosal, Trilisate*
Dosage: 2,000 to 3,000 mg per day in 2 or 3 doses

Choline salicylate (liquid only)
Brand name: *Arthropan*
Dosage: 3,480 mg or 20 ml per day in several doses

Magnesium salicylate
Prescription: *Magan, Mobidin, Mobogesic*
Non-prescription: *Arthritab, Bayer Select, Doan's Pills,*
Dosage: 2,600 to 4,800 mg per day in 3 to 6 doses

Salsalate
Brand names: *Amigesic, Anaflex 750, Disalcid, Marthritic, Mono-Gesic, Salflex, Salsitab*
Dosage: 1,000 to 3,000 mg per day in 2 or 3 doses

Sodium salicylate
Brand name: *Available as generic only*
Dosage: 3,600 to 5,400 mg per day in several doses

COX-2 INHIBITORS

Like traditional NSAIDs, Cox-2 inhibitors help reduce pain and inflammation but are safer for the stomach. Digestive tract studies have shown less stomach damage from COX-2 inhibitors compared to traditional NSAIDs; however, COX-2s have not been used as long as other NSAIDS.

Studies to determine the incidence of side effects and safety continue. In fact, in late 2004 and early 2005, two COX-2s, rofecoxib (*Vioxx*) and valdecoxib *(Bextra)* were withdrawn from the market after several large studies showed increased cardiovascular risk and, in the case of *Bextra*, risk of a serious skin reaction. A long-term study to evaluate the cardiovascular risks of *Celebrex* is underway. In the meantime, the FDA has asked manufacturers of all NSAIDs to include warnings on their labels and to provide consumers with medication guides.

Celecoxib
Brand name: *Celebrex*
Dosage: 200 mg once per day or 100 mg twice per day

ANALGESICS

Unlike NSAIDs, these drugs are used purely for pain relief, not inflammation. So, they may be a more appropriate and safer choice for those with arthritis who suffer pain without inflammation.

Because of its low cost, effectiveness and safety, rheumatologists often recommend the most common analgesic, acetaminophen, first for osteoarthritis. Do not combine acetaminophen with NSAIDs without speaking to your doctor first.

For severe pain, doctors may prescribe opioid analgesics, such codeine or hydrocodone. Sometimes these products also contain acetaminophen, such as oxycodone with acetaminophen (*Percocet*) or proposyphen with acetaminophen (*Darvocet*). If your doctor prescribes one for you, make sure you don't get a double dose of acetaminophen, which can be toxic. Longer-acting opiod analgesics are available, too. Some of these come in pill forms, such as oxycodone ((*OxyContin*); or in a patch that delivers medication through the skin, such as transermal fentanyl (*Duragesic*).

Other than acetaminophen, the drugs listed below have the potential for dependence if used for long periods.

Acetaminophen

Brand names: *Anacin (aspirin-free), Excedrin caplets, Panadol, Tylenol, Tylenol Arthritis*
Dosage: 325 to 1,000 mg every 4 to 6 hours as needed, no more than 4,000 mg per day. For *Tyenol Arthritis*, 1,300 mg every 8 hours as needed; no more than 3,900 mg in 24 hours.
Possible side effects: When taken as directed, acetaminophen is usually not associated with side effects.

Acetaminophen with codeine

Brand names: *Phenaphen with Codeine, Tylenol With Codeine #3*
Dosage: 15 to 60 mg codeine every 4 hours as needed (150 to 600 mg acetaminophen)
Possible side effects: Constipation, dizziness, lightheadedness, sedation, nausea, shortness of breath, vomiting

Hydrocodone with acetaminophen

Brand names: *Dolacet, Hyrocet, Lorcet, Lortab, Vicodin*
Dosage: 2.5 to 10 mg hydrocodone every 4 to 6 hours as needed (acetaminophen portion of medication varies)
Possible side effects: Constipation, dizziness, lightheadedness, mood changes, nausea, sedation, shortness of breath, vomiting, and urinary retention

Morphine sulfate

Brand names: *Avinza, Oramorph ST*
Dosage: For *Avinza*, 30 mg per day in a single dose to star. Doctor may increase dose as necessary; for *Oramorph ST*, 30 to 100 mg every 12 hours
Possible side effects: Constipation, drowsiness, nausea

Drugs Used in Treating Osteoarthritis (cont.)

Oxycodone

Brand names: *OxyContin, Roxicodone, OxyFast, OxyIR (liquid)*

Dosage: For *OxyContin*, 10 mg every 12 hours; for the others, 5 mg every 6 hours as needed

Possible side effects: Constipation, dizziness, drowsiness, dry mouth, headaches, increased sweating, itching of skin, nausea, shortness of breath, vomiting, weakness

Oxycodone with acetaminophen

Brand names: *Percodet, Endocet*

Dosage: 5 mg oxycodone every 6 hours as needed (acetaminophen portion of medication varies depending on whether you are taking pills or capsules.)

Possible side effects: Constipation, dizziness, drowsiness, dry mouth, headaches, increased sweating, itching of skin, nausea, shortness of breath, vomiting, weakness

Propoxyphene hydrochloride

Brand names: *Darvon, PP-Cap*

Dosage: 65 mg every 4 hours as needed, no more than 390 mg per day

Possible side effects: Dizziness, nausea, sedation, vomiting

Propoxyphene with acetaminophen

Brand names: *Darvocet*

Dosage: 50 to 100 mg propoxyphene (325 to 650 mg acetaminophen) every 4 hours as needed, not to exceed 600 mg propoxyphene per day

Possible side effects: Dizziness, nausea, sedation, vomiting

Tramadol

Brand name: *Ultram*

Dosage: 50 to 100 mg every 4 to 6 hours as needed

Possible side effects: Constipation, diarrhea, dizziness, sleepiness, increased sweating, loss of appetite, nausea

Tramadol with acetaminophen

Brand name: *Ultracet*

Dosage: 75 mg tramadol every 4 to 6 hours as needed for up to 5 days (no more than 600 mg per day)

Possible side effects: Constipaton, diarrhea, dizziness, drowsiness, increased sweating, loss of appetite, nausea

TOPICAL ANALGESICS

Topical analgesics are salves, creams and rubs that are applied directly to the skin on the painful area. They should never be taken internally. If you are allergic to aspirin, do not use any topical analgesics containing salicylates, which contain the same medication as aspirin. Never use any topical analgesic in conjunction with a heating pad, because deep burns could result. Read brands' labels for specific dosage information.

Counterirritants

Brand names: *ArthriCare, Eucalyptamint, Icy Hot, Therapeutic Mineral Ice, Menthacin* (also contains capsaicin)

Salicylates

Brand names: *Aspercreme, BenGay, Flexall, Mobisyl, Sportscreme*

Capsaicin

Brand names: *Capzasin-P , Zostrix, Zostrix HP*

HYALURONIC ACID THERAPY

In cases of knee osteoarthritis, hyaluronic acid therapy, or viscosupplements, may be injected directly into the joint to supplement hyaluronic acid, a substance that gives joint fluid its viscosity, or thickness, and that appears to break down in joints with osteoarthritis. The products work as lubricants and relieve pain, but they have not been approved for use on other affected joints.

Possible side effects include pain, fluid collection around the knee, swelling, heat and/or redness at the injection site. These products (except *Euflexxa*) are not recommended for people with joint or skin infections or who are allergic to bird feathers, bird proteins and/or eggs.

Sodium Hyaluronate

Brand name: *Hyalgan, Supartz, Euflexxa*
Dosage: Five 2 ml injections (*Hyalgan*) or 2.5 ml (*Supartz*), one each week for five weeks; For *Euflexxa*, one 2 ml injection per week for three weeks

Hylan G-F 20

Brand name: *Synvisc*
Dosage: 2 ml injections administered once a week for three weeks

Chapter 6

Beyond Drugs:
Other Therapies for Osteoarthritis

Now that you have some background about osteoarthritis, how it affects your body, and drug therapies available to treat your symptoms, we'll take a look at other management strategies that may help you deal with the effects of the disease.

Follow Your Management Plan

You and your doctor will work together to determine an overall treatment plan that meets your specific needs. Your doctor will take into account the severity of your osteoarthritis, the joints that are affected, your age, other medical problems you have, and your lifestyle and daily activities. Non-drug and minimally invasive treatments that still effectively control your symptoms are the preferred options. Fortunately, some very effective osteoarthritis treatments are the least invasive ones – like exercise.

Exercise

Exercise is considered to be the most effective non-drug treatment for reducing pain and improving movement in osteoarthritis. In this section, we'll look at how exercise can help. For more information on specific exercise programs and how to get started, see Chapter 9.

Regular exercise is important for everyone's overall health. It has been shown to reduce the risk of several serious diseases, including hypertension and heart disease. For people with osteoarthritis, exercise is particularly important for increasing your strength and energy level.

You may worry that exercise could harm your joints or cause more pain. But research has shown that people with osteoarthritis can and should exercise. The disease leads to limited motion in your joints, so that you may have trouble moving as much and as comfortably as you did before you had osteoarthritis. Exercise can help you get some of that movement back.

What Kinds of Exercise Are Important?

Three kinds of exercise are important for people with osteoarthritis: range-of-motion, also called flexibility exercises; endurance or aerobic exercises; and strengthening exercises. Each one plays a role in maintaining and improving your ability to move and function.

Don't feel boxed in by these categories. You don't have to follow a boring, regimented program to get the benefits of exercise. The most important thing is that you make an effort to keep moving on a regular basis, no matter what activities you do. The categories are simply guidelines for the types of movements that are helpful for osteoarthritis.

In choosing an exercise program, pick something you enjoy doing and take note of ways you can be more active in your everyday life. Fun activities that you may not think of as exercise – such as gardening, dancing or playing outside with your children or grandchildren – can help you move better and minimize the effects of osteoarthritis.

Here, we'll give you a brief explanation of the exercise types that make up a well-rounded program. Chapter 9 will discuss these types of exercise in more detail and provide some sample moves.

RANGE OF MOTION/FLEXIBILITY

Range of motion refers to the ability to move your joints through the full motion they are designed to achieve. When you have osteoarthritis, pain and stiffness can make it very difficult for you to move certain joints more than just a little bit, which can make even the simplest tasks very challenging.

Range-of-motion exercises include gentle stretching and movements that take joints through their full span. Doing these exercises regularly – ideally every day – can help maintain, and even improve, the flexibility in your joints. Your doctor or physical therapist can show you how to do the exercises properly and safely. For more specific flexibility exercises, see Chapter 9.

AEROBIC/ENDURANCE

Aerobic, or endurance, exercises strengthen your heart and make your lungs more efficient. This conditioning has the added benefit of reducing fatigue, so you have more stamina throughout the day. Aerobic exercise also helps control your weight by increasing the amount of calories your body uses. This type of exercise can help you sleep better and improve your mood.

In Chapter 9, we'll look more closely at specific, safe aerobic exercises and tips for staying motivated.

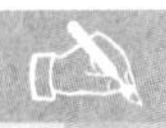

Personally Speaking STORIES FROM REAL PEOPLE

"My 'strategies' [for coping] come from a lifetime of compensation and adaptation. Born with dwarfism and severe scoliosis at a time when medical intervention was limited, I have spent most of my life in a wheelchair and in a world that was much larger than I was, and, until recently, mostly inaccessible.

THERE ARE DAYS WHEN THE SUN SHINES
– RUTH HELEN THOMPSON, STREET, MD

"I completed high school at home, spent a year at a rehabilitation facility and worked as a secretary for 24 years. Adaptations, modifications and attitude have played a major role in my life. My work career ended when I was returning from a visit to my rheumatologist. I had an auto accident that caused a broken arm and a worsening of my arthritis, general strength and endurance. At this point, I am on disability retirement.

"Many of the activities I enjoyed – playing the organ, for example – I can no longer do. I can still do art work during good times. I like to get out and see things and go places. On days when I have pain, I listen to audiobooks, music (especially gospel) and talk on the phone.

"I have learned also that it is all right to be depressed, upset, angry and teary, because there also are days when the sun shines brightly and the birds sing."

STRENGTHENING

Strengthening exercises help maintain and improve your muscle strength. Strong muscles can support and protect joints that are affected by arthritis. In Chapter 9, we'll look at how to strengthen muscles safely with some sample programs.

Weight Control

Body weight plays a significant role in osteoarthritis. As we've already seen in Chapter 1, excess body weight contributes to the development of osteoarthritis. In addition to helping prevent osteoarthritis, controlling body weight is an important treatment for the disease.

If you already have osteoarthritis, maintaining your recommended weight – or losing weight if you are overweight – can lessen pain by reducing stress on your affected joints. Weight loss can especially help your weight-bearing joints, such as hips, knees, back and feet, which already endure a great deal of pressure.

If you need to lose extra body weight, consult your doctor about safe and effective steps you can take. The best way to take off extra pounds and keep them off is by eating fewer calories and increasing your physical activity. You must make sure that you continue to get the proper nutrients to keep your body healthy and that the activities you do won't harm your joints. Your doctor can help you devise an appropriate weight-loss program that will work for you. For more specific information on the importance of nutrition and exercise, see Chapter 10.

Physical and Occupational Therapy

When osteoarthritis affects your ability to do routine tasks, such as household chores, bathing, dressing and walking, you may need the help of a physical or occupational therapist. Usually your doctor will refer you to one of these health professionals.

- Physical therapists work with you on rehabilitation activities, such as restoring muscle strength or improving mobility in affected joints. A physical therapist may design a specific exercise program for you to follow on your own, or he or she may administer pain-management techniques, such as ultrasound, massage or whirlpool therapy.
- Occupational therapists specialize in helping you manage your daily activities more easily. They can show you ways to protect your joints and to perform tasks without putting harmful stress on your joints. Occupational therapists can offer splints or braces to stabilize joints and reduce pain, and they can recommend items, such as kitchen utensils, that are designed to be easier and more comfortable for you to use.

Splints and Braces

Splints and braces, also called orthotic devices, can reduce pain, and protect and support joints affected by osteoarthritis as you go about your daily activities. They can also keep your joints in the correct position during activity and sleep.

Because your joints can become stiff if they stay in one position too long, it is important to use a splint or brace only for a limited amount of time. Be sure that you continue to do appropriate stretching and other range-of-motion activities to keep your joints moving and prevent stiffness.

An occupational therapist can design a splint or brace for just about any joint. Some splints are available over the counter at medical supply stores, but you should get a therapist's advice to help you choose one that fits properly and does what you need it to do.

Talk to your doctor about seeing a physical or occupational therapist if:

- Pain and stiffness are making it hard for you to go about daily activities.
- You want to learn ways to protect your joints from harm or to support unstable joints.

Alternative and Complementary Therapies

Over the past several years, more people have become interested in alternative and complementary therapies. The reasons range from inadequate relief obtained from traditional therapies to an interest in natural treatments. Until recently, the term alternative medicine was used to describe all therapies outside of mainstream Western medicine that were used instead of traditional therapies. Now the more common term is complementary therapies, which refers to unconventional treatments used in conjunction with a traditional treatment plan.

Complementary therapies may:

- ease symptoms, such as pain, stiffness, stress and depression
- improve your outlook and attitude
- work with your conventional therapies to enhance the effects of both

You should not expect complementary therapies to replace the rest of your treatment plan or cure your osteoarthritis. Instead, consider these therapies to be something additional you can do for yourself to take control of your condition.

Always discuss with your doctor any therapy you try. Even so-called "natural" therapies can have side effects or properties that interact with the other medications you're taking. Discussing these therapies gives your doctor the opportunity to keep an eye out for any dangers or side effects you may experience.

For in-depth information on more than 90 alternative and complementary therapies for arthritis, consult the Arthritis Foundation's *Alternative Treatments for Arthritis* (2005), available at bookstores, by calling 800-283-7800 or at www.arthritis.org.

Acupuncture

This centuries-old Chinese therapy is based on the idea that life energy called *qi* (pronounced "chee") flows through the body along clearly defined channels. Illness results when the qi is out of balance. Acupuncture uses very fine needles to stimulate points along those channels to put the qi back in balance.

The scientific explanation for acupuncture's effect is that the inserted needles stimulate the body to release pain-killing chemicals called *endorphins*. Exactly how acupuncture works isn't clear, but it does have real effects.

Some studies indicate that acupuncture may be effective for osteoarthritis treatment. It may help relieve pain when used in conjunction with medications. If you are taking the medications only for pain, and not inflammation, acupuncture may allow you to reduce your dose. A consensus panel convened by the National Institutes of Health concluded that acupuncture can be an effective part of an osteoarthritis treatment plan.

Be sure to choose a qualified acupuncturist who is certified or licensed in your state. Make sure that the acupuncturist uses sterile, disposable needles.

Evaluating Alternative and Complementary Therapies

When you're considering a complementary therapy, be cautious. In your search for relief, you may be willing to try something that holds little promise of helping your condition. In addition to treatments that may help, there are those that can hurt you. Even harmless therapies may cost money, yet deliver no relief.

Be particularly skeptical of therapies that:

- Claim to work by a secret formula
- Say they are a cure or a miraculous breakthrough
- Are publicized in the backs of magazines, over the phone, or through direct mail (bona fide treatments will be reported in medical journals)
- Rely only on testimonials as proof that they work

As you consider an alternative or complementary therapy, keep the following advice in mind:

- Most of these therapies are not regulated. Although drugs and other conventional therapies are monitored and regulated by government agencies like the FDA, such therapies as herbs, supplements and some other alternatives do not have to undergo that scrutiny and are not approved by the FDA. Before you try an alternative treatment, learn as much as you can about it. A good source of information is the National Center for Complementary and

Chiropractic

Chiropractic involves manipulation and manual adjustment of the spine. The practice is based on the idea that dysfunction in the spine can cause problems in other areas of the body.

Chiropractic may provide relief for some people. Manipulation of some joints may help relieve osteoarthritis pain, but joint manipulation of weak or damaged joints can also cause problems. To further investigate the potential benefits of chiropractic, the National Institutes of Health recently established a chiropractic research center to fund research and evaluate the therapy's effectiveness. (For more information, go to http://nccam.nih.gov.)

Alternative Medicine (NCCAM). For a free packet of information on alternative therapies, write to the NCCAM Clearinghouse, P.O. Box 7923, Gaithersburg, MD 20898-8218 or call 888-644-6226.

- Discuss the therapy with your doctor. Your doctor should be informed about any therapy you try, alternative remedy or not. He or she can help you watch for and safeguard against side effects and possible negative interactions with medications you may be taking. Your doctor can answer important questions, such as how the therapy fits into your treatment plan and what precautions you should take.
- If you proceed, do so with caution. Seek out a qualified practitioner. Practitioners of certain therapies are required to be licensed by a state or national board. If that isn't the case, find out about professional societies that provide certification.
- Consider the cost. Some alternative therapies can be costly and they may not be covered by your insurance. Read your policy closely to find out what therapies are covered and under what circumstances.
- Use good judgment. If the practitioner makes unrealistic claims such as, "It will cure your arthritis," or suggests that you discontinue your conventional treatments, consider it a strong warning that something is not right.

(Adapted from *Kids Get Arthritis Too* Newsletter, May/June 1999)

Chiropractic may not be safe for people who have osteoporosis or inflammatory conditions such as rheumatoid arthritis or ankylosing spondylitis. Be sure to tell the chiropractic practitioner about your arthritis and inform your medical doctors about your chiropractic treatment.

Vitamins

Researchers have found that certain vitamins, particularly antioxidants, may help ease certain symptoms of osteoarthritis. Antioxidants help destroy free radicals, which may contribute to diseases. It is generally best to get vitamins from whole foods – such as fresh milk or oranges – rather than supplements, because the body seems to absorb and use whole food nutrients better.

- In studies of animals with osteoarthritis, vitamin C appears to counteract the wearing away of cartilage. And in a 2002 Danish multicenter, double-blind study, 1,000 mg daily of calcium ascorbate – a mix of calcium and vitamin C – significantly reduced osteoarthritis pain in the hip or knee compared to a placebo. However, a 2004 study at Duke University found that high doses – at least 20 times the recommended RDA of 75 to 90 mg – increased the severity of osteoarthritis in guinea pigs. The researchers did see an association between higher levels of vitamin C and increased collagen in knee cartilage. But they also found that vitamin C activated a protein that causes joint deterioration and bony spurs. The researchers concluded that men should not take more than 90 mg of vitamin C supplements and women more than 75 mg per day.
- Research results about vitamin E have been mixed. Some findings show that vitamin E provides some pain relief in people with osteoarthritis; others show no benefits. And one study showed that vitamin E was associated with a lower risk of knee osteoarthritis in Caucasians but not in African-Americans.
- Vitamin D may play a beneficial role in preventing osteoarthritis. Several studies have found that progression of the disease was faster in people who had a low intake of the vitamin. And a 2005 study at Boston University found that vitamin D enhanced bone density in those with knee osteoarthritis.

Herbs and Supplements

If you've seen any magazine or television ads lately, you know that herbs and supplements are a booming business. Herbal remedies are increasingly available to consumers who want help for everything from depression to weight loss and even chronic illnesses like arthritis. People are buying and using herbs and supplements in record numbers. According to a 2005 report by the American Botanical Council, 2004 sales of herbal supplements were almost $258 million.

Herbs and supplements are appealing to people with conditions like arthritis, which have no simple cure. People with arthritis often are frustrated by the lack of relief traditional medicine appears to provide. They hope that "natural" remedies will offer a gentler type of relief for their pain, with fewer unwelcome, dangerous side effects.

Supplements offer the convenience of popping a pill or potion, along with the idea that the organic ingredients pose little danger. But natural doesn't always mean safe. Some people think that supplements – especially herbs – are safer than the synthetic chemicals used in over-the-counter or prescription drugs. But any product with the potential to help could also be strong enough to hurt.

Although some products are unproven and may be dangerous, others may provide some relief. And research shows that certain herbs and supple-

What To Look For

If you decide to try supplements like glucosamine and chondroitin sulfate, take care when choosing a product because supplements are not regulated by the FDA. Here are some other tips to help you:

- Choose products sold by large, well-established companies that can be held accountable for their products.
- Ask your doctor and pharmacist what they recommend.
- Read the label to make sure the ingredient list makes sense to you. Ask your pharmacist for help if you have trouble.
- Choose products that say "standardized" on the label. Also look for "USP" on the label, which means the manufacturer has followed the U.S. Pharmacopoeia's standards. The U.S. Pharmacopoeia is a non-profit organization that establishes standards or supplements and herbs.
- Take note of any side effects you experience and notify your doctor.

ments are helpful in treating some types of arthritis.

Because of the increased use and interest in herbs and other supplements, researchers are continuing to investigate the effects and safety of these compounds to determine if the claims are valid – and if these products have a potential role in osteoarthritis treatment. For many herbs and supplements, there isn't enough scientific evidence to draw a conclusion about their efficacy. Because the remedies are not required to have the same safety and effectiveness testing that pharmaceutical drugs do, it can also be difficult to tell what you are getting.

Consult your doctor before deciding to try an herbal remedy or other supplement, and don't stop your prescribed treatment. Here's a run-down of therapies that may have beneficial effects for osteoarthritis.

Glucosamine and Chondroitin Sulfate

Two supplements that have received attention for arthritis treatment are glucosamine and chondroitin sulfate, both found naturally in the body. Glucosamine is an amino sugar that appears to play a role in the formation and repair of cartilage. Chondroitin sulfate is part of a protein that gives cartilage elasticity.

The two dietary supplements have been used for several years to treat osteoarthritis in dogs and horses, and in Europe to treat osteoarthritis in people. Studies done in Europe have found that people with mild to moderate osteoarthritis who took either supplement reported pain-relief levels similar to those achieved with NSAIDs, although the supplements may take longer to begin working.

The 2005 results from the NIH Glucosamine/Chondroitin Arthritis Intervention Trial (GAIT), the first, large-scale multi-center clinical trial testing the short-term (six months) effectiveness of the supplement in reducing knee osteoarthritis pain suggested this: the combined supplements reduced pain in those with moderate to severe pain but did little for those with mild pain. The upshot: Ask your doctor if glucosamine and chondroitin can play a part in your treatment.

The most common side effects of using glucosamine and chondroitin sulfate are increased intestinal gas and softened stools. Other cautions include:

- Women who are pregnant or who may become pregnant should not take glucosamine and chondroitin sulfate because the effects on unborn children have not been studied.

Herbs and Supplements and Their Uses

Read individual entries on the following pages to learn about the research behind the claims.

Therapy	Symptom					Uses and Comments
	PAIN	STIFFNESS	FATIGUE	INFLAMMATION	ANXIETY/DEPRESSION	
AVOCADO/SOYBEAN OIL	•					For OA
BORON	•	•		•		For RA, OA; may raise estrogen levels
BOSWELLIA	•	•		•		For RA, OA; often used in combinations
CHONDROITIN SULFATE	•	•				For OA
GINGER	•			•		For RA, OA; relieves nausea
GLUCOSAMINE	•	•				For OA
SAM-e	•	•			•	For OA, depression, fibromyalgia

- If you have diabetes, get your blood sugar levels checked frequently because glucosamine is an amino sugar.
- If you take blood-thinning medications or daily aspirin therapy, have your blood-clotting time checked more frequently. Chondroitin sulfate is similar in structure to the blood thinner heparin, and the combination may cause bleeding in some people.
- If you are allergic to shellfish, consult your doctor before taking glucosamine because it is extracted from crab, lobster or shrimp shells. In most cases, however, the allergies are triggered by the proteins in shellfish, and glucosamine is extracted from a carbohydrate called chitin.
- Don't give up your other medications without talking to your doctor.
- Most experts recommend trying the supplements along with your regular medications for six to eight weeks. If you don't experience any change in your symptoms after a few months, then they probably won't work for you.

Other Supplements

Here are some commonly used supplements for osteoarthritis:

- **Avocado/soybean oil**, also called ASU, is a mixture of these two oils that could ease osteoarthritis pain. Four randomized, double-blind European trials done between 1997 and 2002 tested ASU. In three, ASU combined with NSAIDs relieved pain better than placebo plus NSAID. The fourth trial found no difference. In general, the oil reduced the need for NSAIDs and was more effective for knees than for hips.

- **Boron** is a trace mineral found in fruits, vegetables, nuts and dried beans, which helps the body use nutrients like calcium and magnesium. Very few studies have been done on this mineral and arthritis. However, in one study, it eased osteoarthritis symptoms more than placebo. In other studies of large populations that only get 1 mg of boron a day, the incidence of arthritis is 20 to 70 percent. In populations that consume 3 to 10 mg a day, the rate of arthritis is zero to 10 percent.
- **Boswellia** is also known as frankincense. Some studies have found that it may improve blood flow to the joints, decrease pain and increase function in those with osteoarthritis.
- **Ginger** is often taken in the form of tea, extract, or capsules to relieve pain and inflammation. And in fact, several recent studies show that ginger relieves some pain and improves function in those with osteoarthritis.
- **SAM-e**, also called S-adenosylmethionine, is a naturally occurring substance that relieves pain and inflammation in those with osteoarthritis. In fact, research shows that it may relieve pain as well as NSAIDs do without the side effects. Some studies also show that SAM-e helps ease depression. Methionine, an essential amino acid found in protein, converts to SAM-e so eating enough protein is important. And because folic acid is essential for the metabolism of methionine, eating more greens can also increase your body's production of SAM-e.

WORKSHEET: My Treatment Plan

When you are diagnosed with a chronic illness, there are many new things to do. For your treatment plan to be effective, you have to follow it carefully. Write down the treatment plan you've discussed with your doctor and make sure you understand what you need to do and how it should help your osteoarthritis. Discuss any questions you have or changes in your disease with your doctor.

My treatments (include drugs, supplements, exercise, stress management):

____

____

____

How each treatment will help me:

____

____

____

Problems to look out for:

____

____

____

Side effects to call my doctor about:

____

____

____

Lifestyle changes to work on:

____

____

____

Chapter 7

Surgery:
The Benefits and Risks

Most people with osteoarthritis won't need surgery, but when other treatments don't help and there is significant joint damage, surgery may be an option to consider. The decision to have surgery should not be made quickly, and you'll need to discuss it carefully with your doctor and surgeon to determine if it's the right option.

What Are the Benefits of Surgery?

If you have severe joint damage, extreme pain that isn't helped by other treatments, or very limited motion as a result of osteoarthritis, surgery may be necessary. Surgical procedures can provide several benefits, which are explained here.

Improved Movement

The constant wearing away of cartilage can damage your joints, making it more and more difficult for you to move. Losing the ability to move a joint comfortably can have an impact on your activities and your ability to get around and stay independent. Surgery can replace your joint with a new one that makes it easier for you to move and continue some activities you enjoy.

Pain Relief

Osteoarthritis can cause constant pain. For some people, treatments such as physical therapy, exercise and medications don't provide enough pain relief for them to do their usual activities. If other methods don't lessen pain enough, surgery may be something to consider.

Improved Joint Alignment

In some cases, osteoarthritis can cause the joint to become malaligned so that it no longer functions as it should and it looks unusual. In the knees, surgery can help correct or improve this malalignment. But appearance should not be the main reason for having surgery; improved appearance should be a bonus of surgery that is performed to improve movement and relieve pain.

The Risks of Surgery

Although surgery can provide some significant benefits, it is not a perfect solution. As with any surgical procedure there are some important risks to consider in joint surgery.

- Other health problems must be under control. If you have such medical conditions as heart disease or lung problems, the strain of surgery could be too much for you. Infections also must be cleared up before surgery or they could cause serious complications.
- Blood clots can develop. Sometimes people develop blood clots in their legs after surgery. You can reduce this risk by preparing in advance with steps such as taking blood-thinning medications and doing leg exercises to increase circulation before surgery. You should discuss this potential complication with your doctor and surgeon.

Questions To Ask About Surgery

Here are some questions to ask your doctor or surgeon before your surgery:

- What treatments could I have instead of surgery? How successful would they be?
- What's involved in the operation?
- Do you have pamphlets or videos that would give me more information?
- How long will the surgery take?
- What risks are involved? How likely are they to occur?
- What type of anesthesia will be used? What are the risks?
- How much will the surgery help me?
- Will I need to have another operation later?
- How much experience do you have with this procedure?
- Could I talk with another patient who has had this operation?
- What's involved in preparing for the surgery?
- What are the risks if I don't have surgery or if I delay it?

- Being overweight can add extra stress on your heart and lungs during surgery. Excess pounds can also slow your recovery if you have surgery on a weight-bearing joint, such as the hip or knee. If you are overweight, think about the risks carefully and consider losing weight before you decide to go ahead with the operation.

Other Considerations

There are some other important issues to seriously consider before you decide to have surgery.

- Recovery takes time. The operation is just the beginning. After surgery, recovery requires a commitment from you. There will be exercises and a strict treatment plan to follow for at least several weeks after the procedure. Your willingness to put effort into your recovery can make a big difference in how well you recover.
- Surgery is expensive. The cost varies depending on the type of surgery, the hospital, medications and other therapies, special tests and your insurance coverage.

Discuss these concerns with your doctor and insurance company well in advance so you aren't surprised when the bills come.

Types of Surgery

Different types of surgery are performed to help ease severe osteoarthritis symptoms in people who have not had adequate relief from other treatments. These operations typically are performed by orthopaedic surgeons, who are physicians with specialized training in surgery on bones, joints and other parts of the musculoskeletal system. Following are explanations of the different procedures and when they are likely to be used.

Arthroscopy

For this procedure, the surgeon makes a couple of small incisions in the skin and inserts a surgical tool and a viewing device called an arthroscope. This procedure allows the physician to view the inside of the joint to see how much damage there is, and to remove loose growths that may be causing pain. Arthroscopy procedures are done most often on knees and shoulders.

Arthroscopic surgery is less invasive and requires less anesthesia than some other types of surgery. Patients usually recover more quickly from this type of surgery than from standard operations.

Osteotomy

This procedure helps correct bone deformities through cutting and repositioning the bone in patients with malalignment of certain joints and mild osteoarthritis.

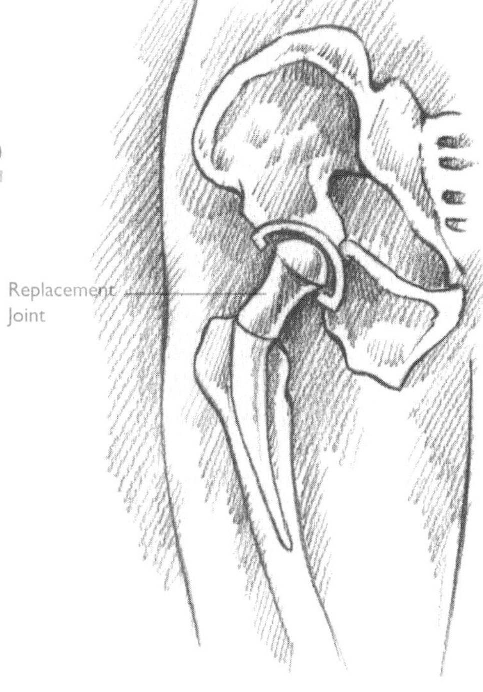

HIP REPLACEMENT

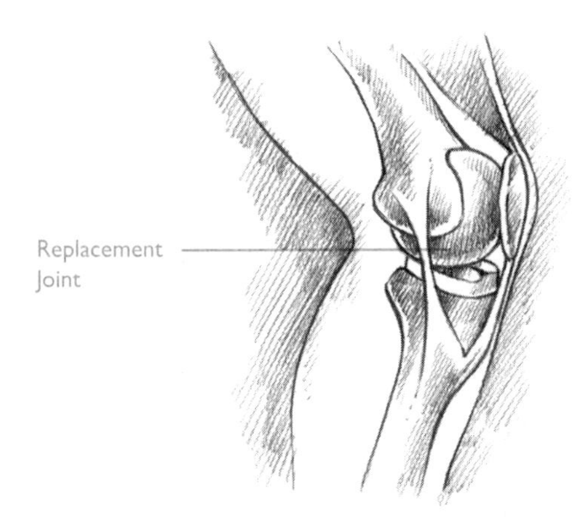

KNEE REPLACEMENT

Osteotomy can correct the forces across the joint, particularly weight-bearing joints of the lower extremities, such as the hip or knee. It occasionally is used for patients who have localized disease involvement with a joint. Osteotomy is useful in patients with unilateral hip osteoarthritis (involvement in only one hip joint), who are too young for a total hip replacement.

Total Joint Replacement

Also called total joint *arthroplasty*, total joint replacement involves removing the damaged bone and joint tissue and replacing them with a new joint made of metal, ceramic and plastic parts. The procedure has been performed widely for many years and is particularly successful for hip and knee joints. Smaller joints also may be replaced, including the shoulder, elbow and knuckle. In 2003, 652,000 joints were replaced in the United States.

There are two options for attaching the replacement joint's components. In one type, the component is fixed with a special type of cement. In the other type, the component has a porous coating that allows bone to grow into the component and hold it in place. The component used is determined by the patient's age and the condition of surrounding bone. Cementless components are typically used in younger people who have a greater amount of hard bone.

Replaced joints last at least 20 years in about 80 percent of people who get them. Both types of replacements, though, can loosen over time and with wear. If the new joint becomes too loose, it may need to be replaced again or revised. According to the National Institutes of Health, about 10 percent of joint replacements need to be revised. It should be noted that there is a greater risk of complications with revision surgeries.

Experimental Therapies

Osteoarthritis once was considered an inevitable part of the aging process. Because cartilage does not have a blood supply, scientists believed that damaged cartilage could not rebuild itself like other tissues, such as skin. Researchers have found that cartilage can grow back after injury; however, the new cartilage usually is weaker and less resilient than the original.

Scientists are studying a procedure in which they encourage cartilage cells to grow in order to repair small defects in human cartilage. Research also is being done to determine whether it's possible to transplant cartilage taken from deceased donors, specifically in the knee. Many approaches remain under study.

PART THREE

Develop a Wellness Lifestyle

Chapter 8

Positive Attitude: Adopting Good Living Strategies

Having a positive outlook about your situation and your life is an important part of living a wellness lifestyle. In addition to taking care of your body, good living means taking care of your mind and spirit. A healthy outlook plays an important role in helping you feel well. There are many ways you can take charge by shaping your attitude and lifting yourself up when you face challenges. This chapter will present some of those methods.

Goal-Setting and Contracting

In assuming responsibility for what you can control, techniques such as goal-setting and contracting can be useful. Although you may not be able to control aspects of osteoarthritis, such as how much pain you experience from day to day, reasonable goals are something you can predict and control.

You can use goal-setting and contracting for many parts of managing osteoarthritis. For example, you can implement a pain-management plan, start an exercise program, change your diet, or make a transition to working from your home.

Chart your course of action by describing a goal in realistic and specific terms. Think of what you would like to do and determine what you can accomplish in the next several weeks or months. If you choose a goal that is too big or that will take too long, you may become discouraged and give up.

Break down your goal into smaller steps or tasks. The steps make your goal more manageable, allow you to track your progress, and also give you a sense of accomplishment. If your goal is to get in better physical shape, for example, you might include these steps:

- Make an appointment with your doctor or a physical therapist to discuss exercise options that may be best for you.

- Find out about specific exercise classes and programs in your area.
- Choose a program and get started.

When you outline steps to your goal, you may find it helpful to create a contract with yourself. A contract is a way of formalizing your goal and the steps you'll take to reach it. Write down your goals, the steps you've determined and specific plans for accomplishing the steps, such as what you will do, how much you will do, when you will do it and how often you will do it. By creating a contract, you also create more of an obligation to fulfill it.

Make your contract realistic. Plan to do something three or four times a week, not every day. Create a contract that you have confidence you can fulfill; for instance, on a scale of zero (completely unsure) to 10

Contract Form

THIS WEEK I WILL: ______________________ **WEEK OF:**______________

For example: This week I will walk around the block before lunch three times.

(WHAT) (HOW MUCH) (WHEN) (HOW MANY)

What

How much

When

How many days

How certain are you *(On a scale of 0 to 10 with 0 being totally unsure and 10 being totally confident)*

Signature

(completely confident), you should have a confidence level of seven or greater that you can meet the terms of the contract. To keep yourself motivated, ask a family member or someone from your health-care team to sign the contract as well.

A Positive Self-Image

Do you believe that you are a worthwhile person with a purpose to your life? Feeling good about yourself is an essential part of being healthy. The chronic pain of osteoarthritis can wear you down, and the stiffness and difficulty moving can make you feel limited in your activities. Work against these negative feelings by focusing on what you can do. Believe in your self-worth and value as a person. This will give your life meaning and help you feel happier and more satisfied.

When chronic pain and stiffness get you down, try some uplifting and pampering activities or anything else that makes you feel good about yourself. Some examples include:

- Get a new hairstyle, spring for a manicure or buy a flattering new piece of clothing.
- Rent the latest comedy or action videos for a movie night.
- Reflect on accomplishments that make you proud.
- Relax with a massage or warm bubble bath.
- Pray or meditate.
- Read an intellectually challenging book.
- Do something to help someone else.
- Write in your journal about the qualities and abilities you like in yourself.
- Learn a new skill.

Self-Talk

Self-talk is the voice in your head that you use to talk to and about yourself. It shapes how you view yourself, your world and your expectations. Self-talk is healthy when it spurs you to achieve success. It can be unhealthy when it focuses on negatives and holds you back.

Unhealthy self-talk comes from responding to situations with erroneous thinking patterns. These patterns can include the following:

- Over-generalizing. You see one event as an ongoing pattern of defeat.
- Thinking in terms of all or nothing. You see things in absolute terms of good and bad or black and white. One experience can color everything.
- Rejecting the healthy experiences. When something good happens, you reject it as a fluke.
- Exaggerating the importance of minor events. You regard minor, random events as having great impact on your life.

- Jumping to conclusions. You assume you know how others are feeling.
- Personalizing unhealthy events for which you aren't responsible. You blame yourself instead of letting others take responsibility for their actions.

To pick out errors in thinking, watch for ways you may focus on the negative or when you use words like can't, always, never, must and if only.

We all sometimes fall into unhealthy self-talk habits. But you can learn to redirect negative thoughts in positive ways. It may take practice, but using positive self-talk can help you overcome challenges. Here's an example:

Unhealthy: I know I should exercise, but I can't. If I did, I know my joints would hurt. I'm too old to get started. I'll never be able to do it.

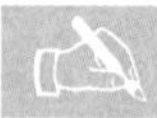

Personally Speaking STORIES FROM REAL PEOPLE

LIVING WELL WITHIN LIMITS

– GLORIA JEWEL LEITNER, ARLINGTON, MA

"The hardest thing for a Peter Pan devotee to admit is, 'I have grown up.' While it's still not beneath my dignity to climb a tree, it is, alas, outside my ability. My hip won't let me attempt many of the activities my tomboy youth allowed me to do.

"There's one big exception, though: bicycling. Arthritis or not, I can still do most of my errands on my bike. With two large baskets in the back, I merrily haul home large grocery bags of food and other parcels.

"My trick is to stow my cane in my backpack when I'm on my bike. It's a fold-up model, and I'm aware that I must make an amusing sight when I hop off my bike – on my good leg, of course – unzip my backpack and whip out my cane! I also like to take a lightweight, three-legged folding chair with me to events such as museum exhibits or walking tours, so I can rest in a comfy seated position.

"What helps me most is doing my physical therapy exercises. I didn't realize how weakened my muscles had become – a major cause of increased pain when I was sitting and lying down. A home regimen of physical therapy exercises has helped me regain much of my muscle strength and dramatically decreased the discomfort.

"Who says you can't partially reverse the effects of a degenerative disease?"

Balancing Act

Consider making a chart to assess the positive and negative influences in your daily life. This chart can help you take a realistic view of what causes your stress. You can also see ways to eliminate or change the negative influences, so that the positives in your life outweigh the negatives. Take a look at the following sample chart, then make your own.

Positives	Negatives
Lunch with friends	Traffic
Support from spouse	Concerns about my health
Gardening	Feeling too busy
Spending time with grandchildren	
Enjoying a good book	

Healthy: Starting to exercise may be difficult, but I can do it if I start slowly.

Have a Sense of Control

Having arthritis can sometimes make you feel as if you have no control over your body or your life. Although you can't choose to get rid of your osteoarthritis, you can choose how you deal with and react to it. Believe in your power to make choices in your life, despite the circumstances that arise.

Feeling a sense of control over what happens to you, instead of feeling helpless and frustrated, will help you to overcome the challenges that life with osteoarthritis can bring. Cultivate that sense of control. Keeping a journal, monitoring your symptoms and following self-care practices, such as exercise and joint protection, are good steps toward taking control of your situation.

Reduce the Negatives

Part of being healthy is having a positive outlook. To foster one, the uplifting influences in your life should outweigh the negative ones.

Think about the many activities and influences in your daily life. Consider making a list of each type so you can compare them. Do your positives outweigh the negatives? Or do you feel so weighed down by the negative ones that you can't enjoy the positives?

WORKSHEET: The Best of Me

List at least 10 qualities or aspects that make you unique, that you like or admire about yourself, and/or that make you attractive (include at least one or two physical attributes).

1	
2	
3	
4	
5	
6	
7	
8	
9	
10	

Now think carefully about the negative activities and influences you encounter. Can you find ways to turn them into positives or eliminate them from your life? This may not work for everything on your list, but give it a try. See if you can either change your thinking about the influence, change some aspect to make it positive, or take it out of your life.

At the same time, try to find ways to maximize the positive aspects of your life. Include more of them, if you can, or figure out how to focus more on the things that make you feel good. Spend less time and energy thinking about the items on the negative list, and you will shift weight over to the positive side.

Have a Sense of Purpose

One of the best ways to keep up a positive outlook and self-image is to remain active – in exercise and in life. Although osteoarthritis may limit some of your movements, don't let it keep you from interacting with friends and doing activities you enjoy.

Withdrawing from activity because of pain and physical limitations only narrows your world more. You can stay engaged and active by continuing the activities you can. If an activity becomes too difficult for you, find a way to modify it or replace it with something you'd like to learn. Participating in social and other activities will make you feel better than isolating yourself.

You may feel that you are always the one who needs extra help or support. But feeling needed and helpful makes those who help you feel important. Try to find ways that you can be helpful and supportive to someone who needs your help.

Activities can lift your spirits and help you keep going when you're in pain. They provide something to look forward to and are great sources of social support. Here are some ways to keep a sense of purpose and stay active:

- Volunteer your time and talents to an organization with a mission that's important to you, such as the Arthritis Foundation.
- Offer to help a friend or a child who could use assistance or a little extra attention.
- Find an outlet for your creative energies – like a hobby you enjoy, an art class, or a friend to cook with (also great way to get help preparing meals).
- If you aren't able to work full time or no longer want to, consider a low-pressure position where you can work a handful of hours a week. It will give you a sense of productivity and an opportunity to interact with co-workers, without the pressure or obligation of full-time work.

The Arthritis Foundation Self-Help Program:

A Tool for Gaining Control

Developed in 1979, the Arthritis Foundation Self-Help Program is a pioneering program that helps people with arthritis learn skills to help them control their disease. Researchers Kate Lorig, RN, DrPH, and James Fries, MD, created the six-week program, which includes information on exercise, pain relief, doctor-patient communication and joint protection.

Perhaps most important, the program teaches self-efficacy. Because of the challenges osteoarthritis can bring, self-efficacy is an important part of managing the disease without feeling overwhelmed by it.

The Arthritis Foundation Self-Help Program is taught by the Arthritis Foundation in local chapter offices, hospitals and community centers. For more information on the availability in your area, contact your local Arthritis Foundation chapter or call 800-568-4045.

Have a Sense of Humor

A healthy dose of laughter is a great way to cultivate positive energy. Research has found that humor can ease the pain and frustration of chronic illness. It helps you see the brighter side of life, and helps you let go of feelings of frustration or depression. Here are some ways to make humor part of your everyday routine:

- See the funny side of life. When you're feeling down, try to see the humorous side of frustrating situations. Try making a joke about the difficulty to lighten your outlook.
- Start a humor collection. Take note of what makes you laugh and collect articles, quotes, comic strips, videos, books or anything that you find funny. When feelings of depression creep up on you, use your collection to help yourself start smiling again.
- Surround yourself with humor. Place fun reminders near your desk at work or in your home so you find something funny when you need it – daily.

Chapter 9

Getting Fit:
Exercise Tips for Osteoarthritis

Regular exercise is important for everyone. It improves cardiovascular fitness so that your heart and lungs work more efficiently and keeps your muscles and bones strong to ward off conditions like osteoporosis. For people with osteoarthritis, exercise is an essential part of an overall treatment plan. It helps loosen stiff joints, keeps muscles strong to support joints and is key to a successful weight-loss program, reducing stress on joints, as explained in Chapters 6 and 10.

The Benefits of Exercise

Although you may know that exercise is good for you and important for managing osteoarthritis, you may still be hesitant to start an exercise program. Perhaps you've never exercised regularly and you're not sure how to get started. Maybe you're afraid that exercising will increase the pain in your already sore joints and cause more joint damage. You may think that exercise is too difficult because you can no longer move your body the way you could before osteoarthritis. Or, you may simply think exercise sounds boring.

Dispel those thoughts. The truth is, you don't have to be an athlete or have your body in perfect condition to exercise and gain its benefits. As you'll see in this chapter, many forms of exercise can accommodate a wide range of abilities. You can start slowly with activities you are comfortable with and capable of doing, then gradually increase your levels as you feel capable.

Exercise isn't a competition. Every bit you do benefits your body and mind – and will help protect your painful joints.

You may need to adjust your mindset a bit. Don't think of exercise as work or as a chore. Moving your body should be fun. Think of exercise as recreation and of your workouts as time you carve out each day to enjoy yourself and move your body.

Why Exercise?

No matter who you are, some kind of exercise is good for you, and research has shown that it can be especially helpful if you have osteoarthritis. The disease process – and the damage it causes – may lead to limited joint range of motion, decreased muscle strength and endurance, and general deconditioning. Exercising – even a little bit – is an important way that you can prevent some of these negative effects.

Research also shows that people with osteoarthritis have lower-than-normal cardiovascular fitness for their age and gender. Some studies have found that people with osteoarthritis who walked on a treadmill stopped as a result of fatigue and lack of conditioning – not pain. A modest exercise program will give your body the flexibility and stamina it needs to do the everyday activities you enjoy.

Studies suggest that losing weight, strengthening the quadriceps muscles (located in the thighs) and improving general fitness can reduce the effects of osteoarthritis on your body and prevent disability. Exercise can boost your weight-loss program, and can help reduce pain, fatigue and depression.

Benefits of Exercise

If you're not sure how exercise can help you, here's a sampling of ways exercise benefits people with osteoarthritis. Exercise can:

- Reduce stiffness
- Strengthen muscles around your joints
- Maintain strength and health of cartilage and bone
- Improve your ability to do daily activities
- Improve your overall health and fitness
- Reduce depression
- Give you more energy
- Control your weight
- Lower stress and tension
- Release endorphins, the body's natural pain-killers
- Improve sleep
- Improve your self-esteem and sense of well-being
- Reduce fatigue

What if I Don't Exercise?

When you're in pain, the last thing you may want to do is move. But if you don't exercise and move your joints, you'll feel worse. Not moving your joints makes them more stiff and painful. People who are in pain tend to guard the painful areas and reduce activities. This makes the muscles supporting the joints too weak to protect the joint or compensate for the joint's limited motion.

Daily activities made more difficult because of arthritis may become impossible to do if you don't keep your joints and muscles in shape through exercise. Not being able to do activities can make you feel more limited by the disease, leading to lowered self-esteem and feelings of depression, which in turn can add to your pain.

People with osteoarthritis may keep their joints bent in one position because it is more comfortable. If you keep joints in one position too long, however, you may lose the ability to straighten them. Exercise gets you in the habit of moving your joints so that doesn't happen.

Because you have arthritis, keeping your muscles as strong as possible is very important. The stronger the muscles and other tissues around the joints, the better they can support and protect them – especially those that are weakened or damaged by arthritis. Another important benefit is that exercise can help reduce your pain so that you may have less need for pain-relieving drugs.

Before You Get Started

When you have osteoarthritis, you need to take care of the joints affected by the disease. Part of that care is learning from a health professional – such as your doctor or a physical therapist – how to do exercises correctly to prevent injury and pain.

Before starting any exercise program, find out which exercises are appropriate for you and what precautions you should take because of your medical condition. Ask about specific activities or movements you should not do. If you don't know where to find an exercise program, ask your physician or other health professional for resources, such as recommended exercise classes and pamphlets with diagrams of proper techniques and sample exercises. Also, your local chapter of the Arthritis Foundation can point you to appropriate exercise programs. You can locate your local chapter by calling 800-568-4045 or visiting www.arthritis.org.

Getting Started and Staying Motivated

The idea of starting an exercise program can be intimidating, particularly if you've never been active. Start slowly. If you feel unable to maintain a regular, strenuous workout at first, do whatever you can. For instance, try to sustain a normal activity just a little longer. As you become stronger and your endurance increases, you will be able to exercise longer and more strenuously.

The toughest part of exercise is getting started. But the effort you put into starting and maintaining a regular exercise program will reward you with better health, less pain and improved outlook. Once you begin to enjoy such benefits, you will also have an easier time sticking to your exercise plan. Your body will become more conditioned, and you may even begin to look forward to your workouts.

Here are some strategies that can help you stay motivated to continue your exercise program:

- Set a realistic exercise goal and sign a contract with yourself, witnessed by a family member, friend, or exercise buddy. Write down what you plan to do and when you plan to do it.
- Exercise at the same time each day so that it becomes a part of your routine. Link the time to something else. For example, after your morning shower, or before lunch.
- Stay in the habit by doing some exercise every day. On days when you have more pain or don't feel motivated, make some effort – even if you just do some gentle stretching or range-of-motion exercises.
- Vary your routine. Some exercises, such as range-of-motion or strengthening exercises, are repetitive and can be boring. Try doing them to music or with a friend or family member. Rotate other exercises. For example, you could walk three days a week, swim twice a week and attend an arthritis exercise class twice a week.
- Evaluate your progress and enjoy your successes. For instance, your doctor may notice increased range of motion, decreased stiffness or improved gait. You probably will see other benefits, such as less fatigue, less pain and decreased stress.

Choosing the Right Exercises

When you're getting started, you may not know exactly where to begin and which exercises are appropriate for you. Discuss options with your doctor and other health-care professionals, and make sure that your routine contains the three basic parts of a complete program outlined in this chapter: flexibility, strengthening and aerobic activities. Arrange your program to include these three types of exercise in ways that match your physical capabilities and your fitness goals.

Flexibility/Range-of-Motion Exercises

Flexibility exercises (also called range-of-motion or stretching exercises) keep your muscles stretched and your joints moving freely. Think of these exercises as the foundation of your program because flexibility is necessary for comfortable movement during exercise and daily activities. Flexibility exercises also reduce the risk of sprains and strains.

Flexibility exercises should be done gently and smoothly, usually every day. You may be familiar with this type of exercise as a "warm up," because these moves are recommended before performing any vigorous type of exercise.

If you have been inactive for a while, or if you have stopped exercising temporarily because of your arthritis, these exercises are a good way to begin your fitness program. Start by building up to a daily routine of

Perceived Exertion Scale

During aerobic activity, it's important to measure how hard you are working. One way is to use the Perceived Exertion Scale: rate how hard you are working on a scale of zero (doing nothing) to 10 (working so hard that you can't keep it up for long). If you are new to exercising or have significant limitations, begin at a very light to fairly light level (2-3). Aim for reaching a moderate to hard intensity (4-7) eventually.

- **0** Nothing (such as lying down)
- **1** Very, very light (almost nothing)
- **2** Very light
- **3** Fairly light
- **4** Moderate (still light but starting to work a little more)
- **5** Moderate (still comfortable but harder)
- **6** Moderate (getting to be somewhat hard)
- **7** Somewhat hard
- **8** Hard
- **9** Very hard
- **10** Very, very hard (couldn't do this for more than a few seconds)

The Talk Test

The talk test is a simple way to tell if you're exercising at an appropriate aerobic level. You should be able to carry on a conversation while exercising, without feeling out of breath. If you're unable to talk, slow down until you're working at a comfortable level.

Any exercise that uses your large muscles in a continuous, rhythmic activity can be an aerobic workout. Some examples include walking, bicycling, aerobic dance and water aerobics. The signs that you are exercising at an aerobic conditioning level are:

- Increased heart rate
- Increased breathing rate
- Increased body temperature or sweating

15 minutes of flexibility exercises. When you are able to do 15 continuous minutes, you should have the mobility and endurance needed to begin adding strengthening and aerobic exercise to your program. If stiffness is a problem for you, consider taking a hot bath or shower before exercising to help "loosen up" joints.

Some sample flexibility exercises are included at the end of this chapter.

Strengthening Exercises

Exercises that increase muscle strength and endurance are the second important component of your fitness program. Joint swelling, pain, and lack of use can weaken muscles. If you have arthritis, strong muscles are particularly important to help absorb shock, support joints and protect you from injury. You need strong muscles to climb stairs, walk safely, lift and reach.

Studies have found that among people with osteoarthritis, the ability to extend the knee often decreases in both the knee affected by the disease and the unaffected knee. In addition, reduced strength in the lower body is linked with increased disability from osteoarthritis. Fortunately, research has also shown that strengthening muscles in the knee, hip and ankle leads to improved balance and increased independence.

Strengthening exercises (also called *resistance exercises*) make your muscles work harder by adding weight or resistance to movement. Flexibility exercises can become strengthening exercises when you increase the speed, increase the number of repetitions, or add weight (resistance) to the exercise. The two types of strengthening exercises are isometric and isotonic exercises. During isometric exercises, you strengthen the muscles by tightening them without moving your joints. Isotonic exercises are just the opposite: You strengthen the muscles by moving your joints.

The goal of a strengthening program is to overload your muscles just enough so they adapt by becoming stronger. This can be done by adding hand-held or wrap-around weights, using elastic bands, or using the weight of your body. You can use weight machines or the resistance of water in pool exercises. But avoid over-loading muscles so much that they are sore and stiff for a day or two after exercising.

Recommended Heart-Rate Ranges

AGE	HEART RATE RANGE (60% - 75% of Age-Predicted Maximum Heart Rate)	10-SECOND COUNT
20	120 – 150	20 – 25
25	117 – 146	19 – 24
30	114 – 143	19 – 24
35	111 – 139	18 – 23
40	108 – 135	18 – 23
45	105 – 131	17 – 22
50	102 – 128	17 – 21
55	99 – 124	16 – 21
60	96 – 120	16 – 20
65	93 – 116	15 – 19
70	90 – 113	15 – 19
75	87 – 109	14 – 18
80	84 – 105	14 – 18
85	81 – 101	13 – 17
90	78 – 98	13 – 16

If you have active inflammation or if your doctor has warned you to protect certain joints, check with a therapist about which strengthening exercises are best and safest for you. If you have been inactive, start by doing 15 minutes of flexibility exercises before you attempt the strengthening ones. When you begin, you'll want to start with no weights or very light weights, and gradually add weight as you feel stronger. Sample exercises are illustrated at the end of this chapter.

Aerobic (Cardiovascular) Exercises

Aerobics include a wide variety of physical activities, not just the popular classes set

Walking Progression

The following suggestions of how much to increase the length of your walks can help you get started with appropriate goals in mind. When you can walk for a total of 10 minutes at a time (including warm-up and cool-down), follow this chart to build your fitness program. If you can already walk for longer than 10 minutes at a time, enter the chart at your current level and progress from there.

WEEK	TIME DURATION PER WALKING SESSION*	FREQUENCY PER WEEK
1	10 minutes	3-5 times
2	15 minutes	3-5 times
3	20 minutes	3-5 times
4	25 minutes	3-5 times
5	30 minutes	3-5 times
6	30-35 minutes	3-5 times
7	30-40 minutes	3-5 times
8	30-45 minutes	3-5 times
9	30-50 minutes	3-5 times

10 and onward: Keep your walks at 30 to 60 minutes per session, 3 to 5 times per week. Gradually increase your intensity until you are in the moderate range (if you are not doing so yet).

* Includes warm-up and cool-down, but not stretching.

For an in-depth guide on starting and maintaining a walking program for people with arthritis, look for the Arthritis Foundation's book *Walk With Ease* at bookstores, at www.arthritis.org or by calling 800-283-7800.

to jazzy beats offered at most health clubs. Also known as endurance or cardiovascular exercises, aerobic exercises use the body's large muscles in cadenced, continuous motions. Swimming, walking, swing dancing, riding a bicycle and even raking leaves are all aerobic exercises.

Aerobic exercise is the third component of your exercise routine. It makes your heart, lungs, blood vessels and muscles work more efficiently. Aerobic exercise is key to achieving overall health. It reduces your risk of developing diabetes, heart disease and high blood pressure. By making aerobic exercise a regular part of your routine, you may improve endurance and sleep, reduce the effects of stress, strengthen bones and control weight.

You should include some type of aerobic exercise three to four times in your weekly fitness routine. Aim to work within your target heart rate – usually about 60 to 85 percent of your maximum heart rate – for 30 minutes each session.

If you find that you cannot exercise continuously for 30 minutes, progress to this level slowly. Begin by gradually increasing your activity for five minutes, continue with five minutes of activity in your recommended heart range (see chart, page 91), then decrease activity for five minutes. Once you have mastered this routine, increase the length of activity in your target range.

- **Walking.** This is an excellent type of aerobic exercise for almost everyone. Walking requires no special skills and is inexpensive. You will need a good pair of supportive walking shoes, however. You can walk almost anytime and anywhere. Many towns now have mall walking clubs, providing a safe place to exercise no matter what the weather is like outside.
- **Water exercise.** Swimming and exercising in warm water are especially good for stiff joints and sore muscles. Water helps support your body while you move your joints through their range of motion. Swimming is highly recommended because little stress is placed on your joints. In many cities, the Arthritis Foundation offers an aquatics exercise program designed for people with arthritis. Call your local Arthritis Foundation chapter or check with your local YMCA or health club to see if this class is offered.
- **Bicycling.** Cycling on a stationary bicycle is a good way to get aerobic exercise without placing much stress on your hips, knees or feet. Some stationary bicycles allow you to exercise your upper body as well. When beginning, try not to pedal faster than five to10 miles per hour. As you become more fit, you can increase

your speed and/or add resistance to your workout. If you have osteoarthritis of the knee, you may wish to consult your doctor or physical therapist to determine if bicycling is an acceptable exercise for you.

A Note About Pain

You may be afraid to exercise too vigorously for fear of causing pain or damage to your joints. This is a common concern for many people with osteoarthritis. Learning to tell the difference between the pain you experience from sore muscles after exercising and the pain caused by overuse or inflammation of joints is important.

Sore muscles are usually the result of overstretching or overuse after a long period of inactivity. This type of pain usually begins several hours after exercising and may continue for 24 to 36 hours.

If you experience muscle soreness, spend more time doing flexibility or warm-up exercises before proceeding to more vigorous activity. You may want to scale back your program until your muscles become more accustomed to exercise and more gradually increase your workout.

Overuse of joints is usually signaled by pain or swelling. If you notice these symptoms, treat the joint by elevating and resting it, and by using ice packs to keep swelling down. Review your exercise program with your doctor or therapist and modify it to avoid further injury to the joint.

One further note about pain: Exercise is one of the most effective nondrug tools you can use to reduce pain associated with arthritis. So exercise sensibly, but do exercise.

How to Know If You're Doing Too Much

When beginning an exercise program, it is important to start slowly and increase your activity level gradually. Watch for the signs that you may be doing too much:

- Increased pain that lasts for more than an hour after exercise
- Increased feelings of weakness
- Excessive tiredness
- Decreased range of motion

Don't Go It Alone

Most people who exercise on their own find it hard to stay motivated and keep going. It helps if you can exercise with at least one other person. Two or more people can keep each other motivated, and joining a class can give you a feeling of shared goals and camaraderie.

Most communities offer a variety of exercise classes, including programs for people with arthritis, people over 50 and people who need adaptive exercises. The Arthritis Foundation sponsors exercise programs developed for people with arthritis. For information, contact your local chapter or branch office. Programs also are available through local YMCA organizations, health clubs, hospital-sponsored fitness facilities, community colleges, parks and recreation departments and senior centers.

If you would like to join a community exercise class or health club, look for one

Getting Yourself To the Next Step

Making exercise a regular part of your life can be a challenge. As with other major lifestyle changes, it requires that you go through changes in your thinking. Consider where you are in the following stages of change and how to get yourself to the next step.

1. You don't understand how exercise can help you. Have your posture or muscle strength checked at a health fair or screening program. A health professional can help you identify areas for improvement and potential benefits from exercise.
2. You know exercise is good for you and you're thinking about starting. Try to connect exercise with something you'd like to be able to do, like playing with your grandchildren or going on a hike. Look at exercise as a way of making these activities possible. Find other people who exercise and get ideas from them about exercising successfully.
3. You're getting ready to start an exercise program. Learn proper exercise techniques so you can prevent pain and injury. Talk to your doctor about appropriate forms of exercise for you. Make a plan by signing up for a class or sketching out a walking program. Set exercise goals for yourself.
4. You've started exercising. Make it a habit. Concentrate on good exercise techniques, such as warming up and cooling down, to prevent pain that could discourage you later. Follow good form and gradually increase your exercise level as you work toward your goal.
5. You've been exercising for six months or more. Great! Keep it up. Set new goals and vary your routine or try new activities so you don't get bored.

(Adapted from *Arthritis Today*, Jan-Feb '99 issue)

that offers classes that meet your needs. Staff members should be qualified or certified by a professional organization, with training or experience in teaching exercise for people with arthritis or other special needs. The facilities should be physically accessible, including the bathroom and changing areas. In addition, make sure you feel comfortable with the staff and other members. Make sure instructors are willing to listen and respond to your concerns about special needs or modifications.

Sample Exercises

Here are some sample range-of-motion and strengthening exercises that you can use in either a warm-up or a cool-down. Select the exercises that are best for you, avoiding those that stress already painful areas. We have excerpted the exercises from the Arthritis Foundation Exercise Program. To purchase copies of the DVD of the program, *Take Control With Exercise,* call 800-283-7800 or shop online at www.arthritis.org.

NECK EXERCISES

Purpose: Increase neck movement; relax neck and shoulder muscles; improve posture.

Precautions: Do these exercises slowly and smoothly. If you feel dizzy, stop the exercise. If you have had neck problems, check with your doctor before doing these exercises.

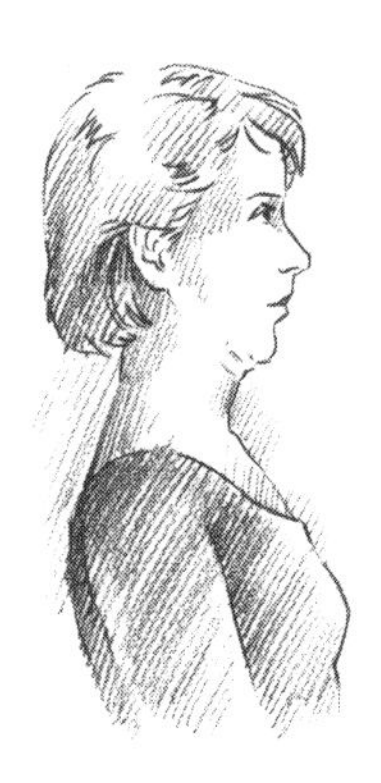

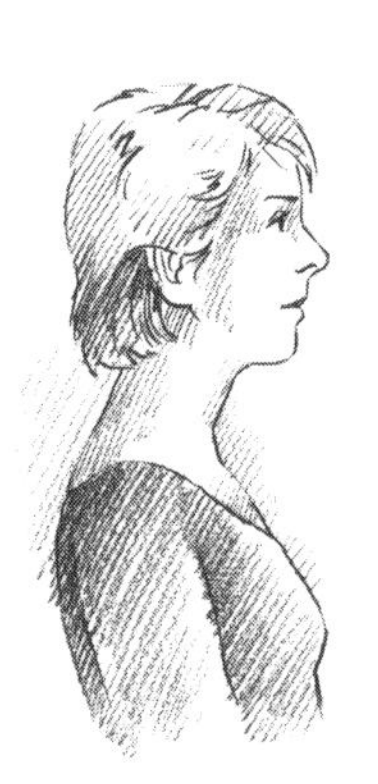

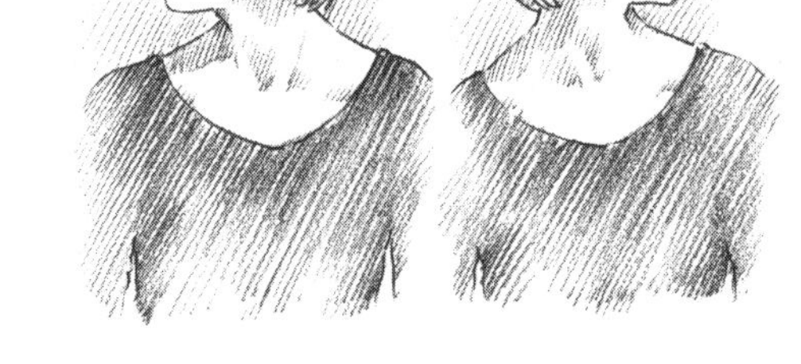

1. CHIN TUCKS

Pull your chin back as if to make a double chin. Keep your head straight – don't look down. Hold three seconds. Then raise your neck straight up as if someone was pulling straight up on your hair.

2. HEAD TURNS (Rotation)

Turn your head to look over your shoulder. Hold three seconds. Return to the center and then turn to look over your other shoulder. Hold three seconds. Repeat.

SHOULDER EXERCISES

Purpose: Increase mobility of the shoulder girdle (the bony structure that supports your upper limbs); strengthen muscles that raise shoulders; relax neck and shoulder muscles.

Precautions: If the exercise increases pain, stop and consult with your physician.

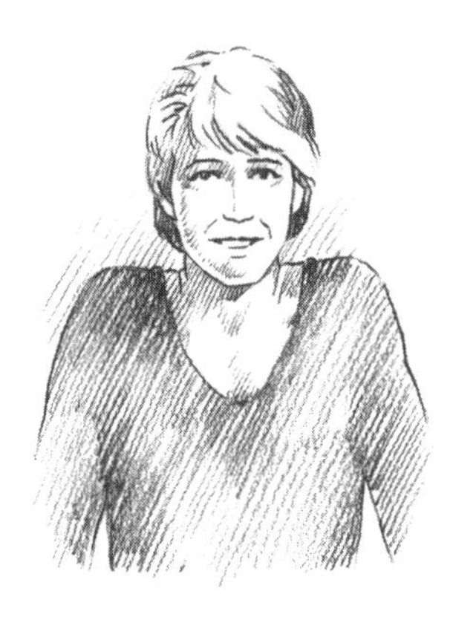

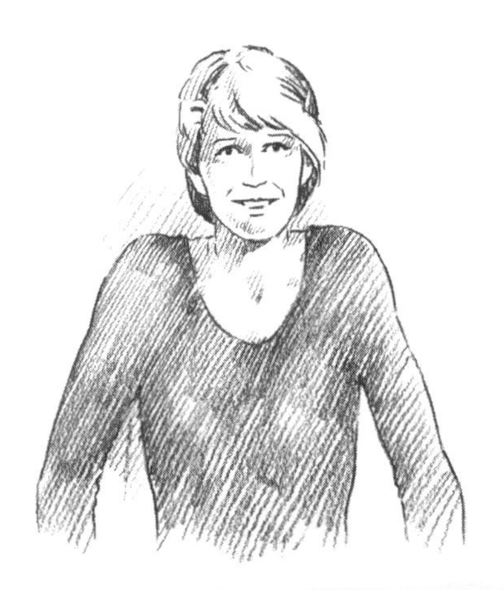

3. SHOULDER CIRCLES

Lift both shoulders up, move them forward, then down and back in a circling motion. Then lift both shoulders up, move them backward, then down and forward in a circling motion.

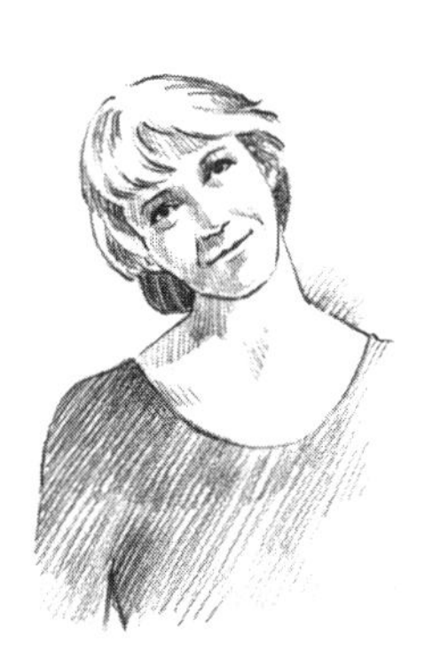

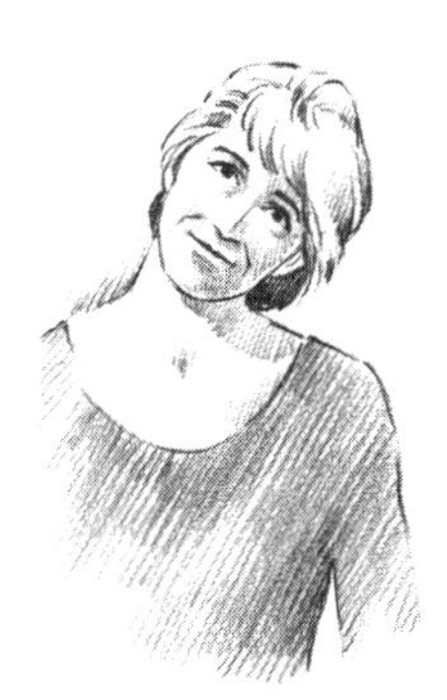

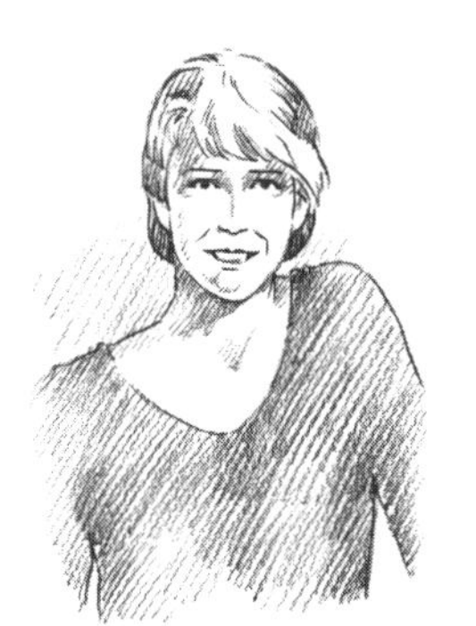

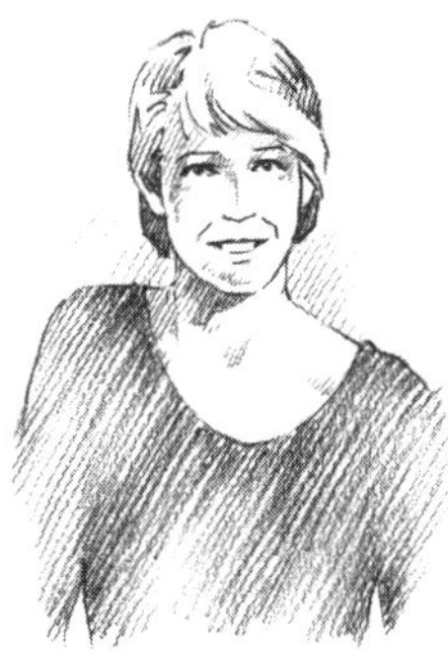

4. HEAD TILTS

Focus on an object in front of you. Tilt your head sideways toward your right shoulder. Hold three seconds. Return to the center and tilt toward your left shoulder. Hold three seconds. Do not twist head but continue to look forward. Do not raise your shoulder toward your ear.

5. SHOULDER SHRUGS

(A) Raise one shoulder, lower it. Then raise the other shoulder. Be sure the first shoulder is completely relaxed and lowered before raising the other.
(B) Raise both shoulders up toward the ears. Hold three seconds. Relax. Concentrate on completely relaxing shoulders as they come down. Do not tilt the head or body in either direction. Do not hunch your shoulders forward or pinch shoulder blades together.

ARM EXERCISES (Shoulders and Elbows)

Purpose: Increase shoulder and/or elbow motion; strengthen shoulder and/or elbow muscles; relax neck and shoulder muscles; improve posture.

Precautions: If you have had shoulder or elbow surgery, check with your surgeon before doing these exercises. These exercises are not advised for people with significant shoulder joint damage, such as unstable joints or total cuff tears.

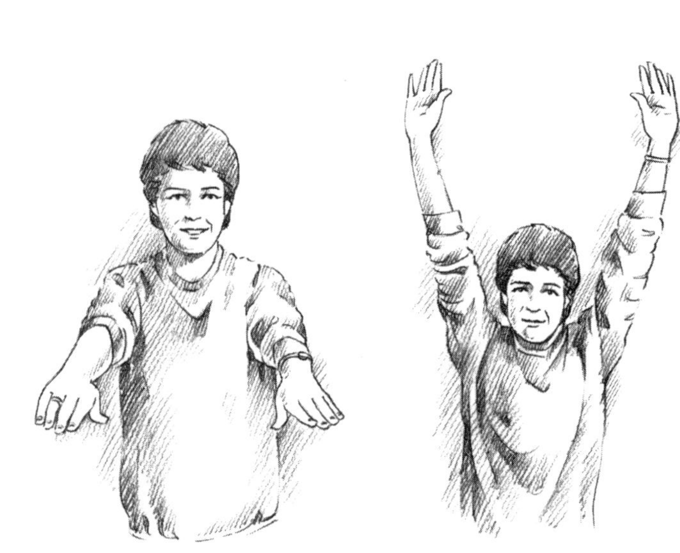

6. FORWARD ARM REACH

Raise one or both arms forward and upward as high as possible. Return to your starting position.

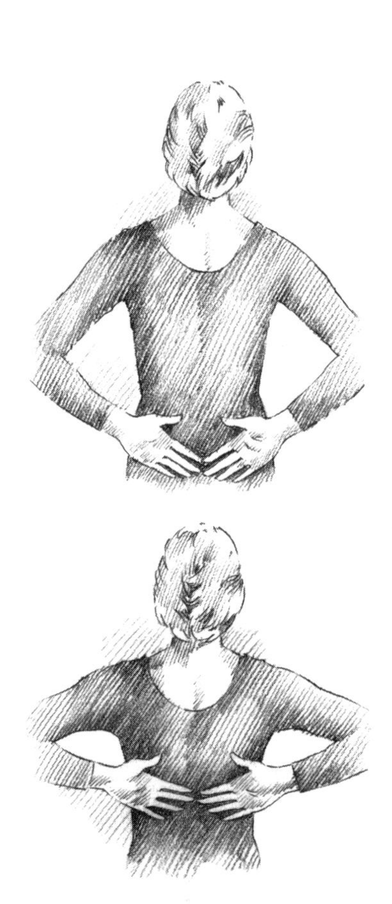

7. SELF BACK RUB

While seated, slide a few inches forward from the back of your chair. Sit up as straight as possible; do not round your shoulders. Place the back of your hands on your lower back. Slowly move them upward until you feel a stretch in your shoulders. Hold three seconds, then slide your hands back down. You can use one hand to help the other. Move within the limits of your pain. Do not force.

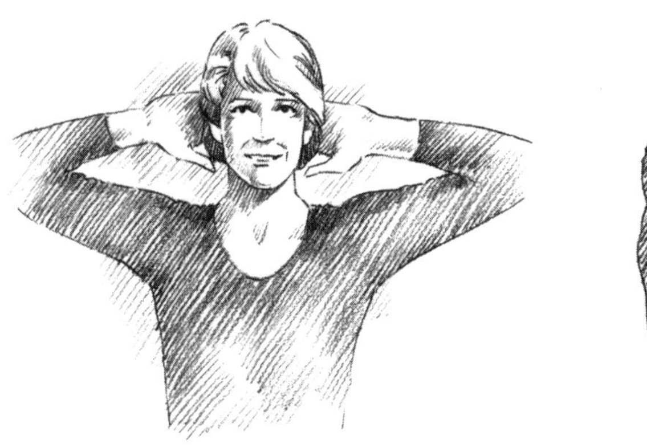
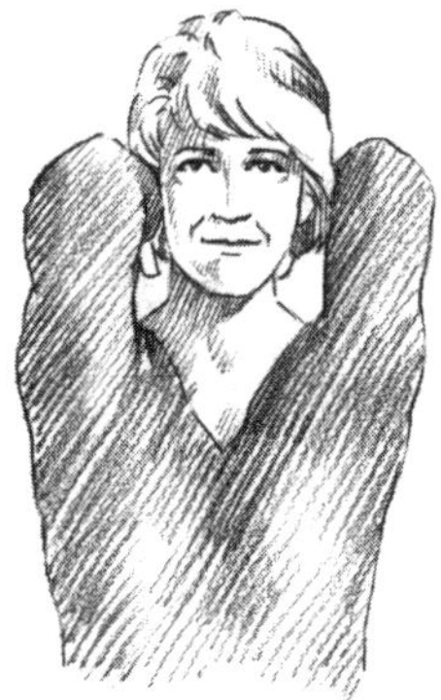

8. SHOULDER ROTATOR

Sit or stand as straight as possible. Reach up and place your hands on the back of your head. (If you cannot reach your head, place your arms in a "muscle man" position with elbows bent in a right angle and upper arm at shoulder level.) Take a deep breath in. As you breathe out, bring your elbows together in front of you. Slowly move elbows apart as you breathe in.

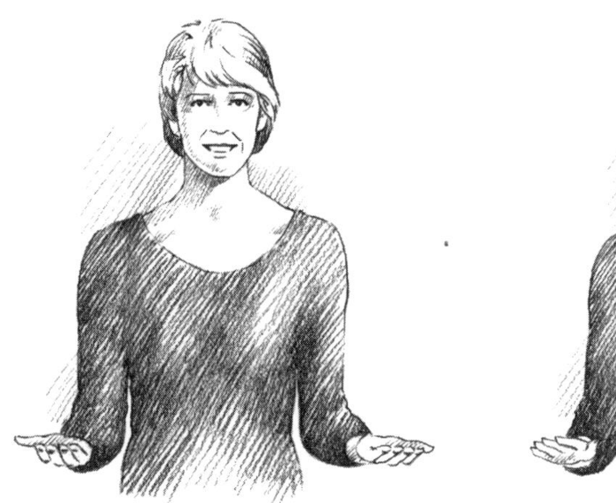
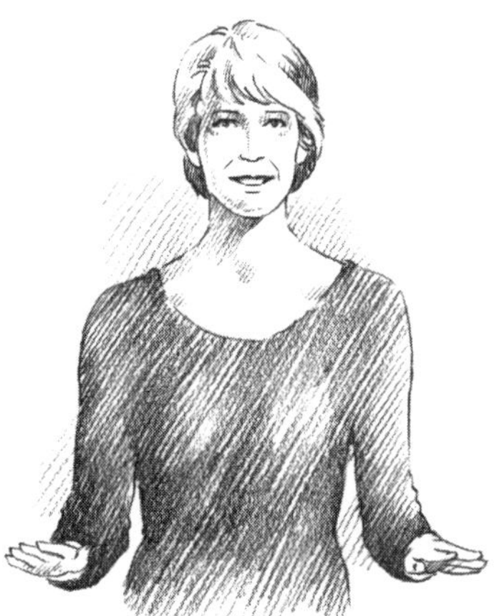

9. DOOR OPENER

Bend your elbows and hold them in to your sides. Your forearms should be parallel to the floor. Slowly turn forearms and palms to face the ceiling. Hold three seconds and then turn palms slowly toward the floor.

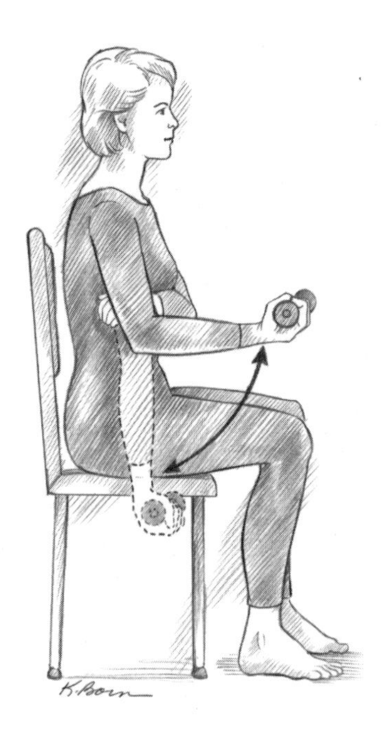

10. BICEPS CURL

Sit in a chair, feet on the floor. Hold a one-pound weight in your right hand, letting your arm hang at your side. Bring your left arm across your chest, resting the back of your right arm on your left fist. Slowly bend your elbow, turning your right forearm toward the front of your shoulder. Your palm should be facing your shoulder. Pause, then lower your arm to the count of three. Repeat on the left side.

11. OVERHEAD TRICEPS

Sit in a chair, holding a one-pound weight in your right hand. Bring your right arm above your head, stopping when the inside of your elbow is above your right ear. Support your right upper arm with your left hand. Slowly bend your right elbow, lowering the weight to your right shoulder. Straighten your elbow to the count of three, pause, then lower it back to your shoulder. Repeat with the left arm.

(These two exercises adapted from *Arthritis Today*)

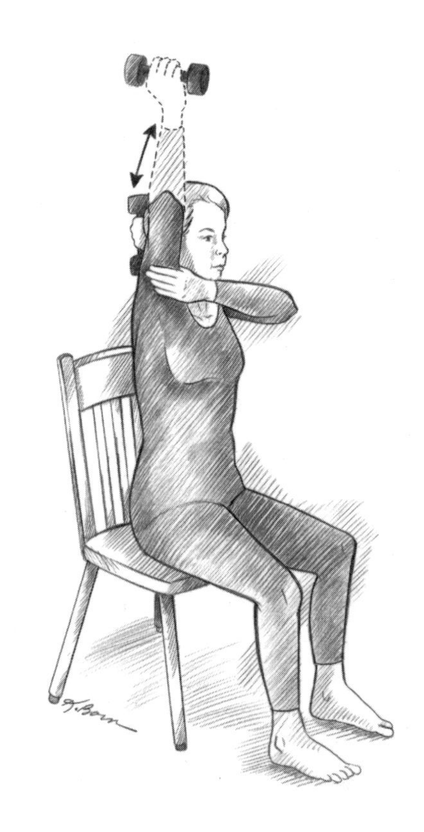

WRIST EXERCISES

Purpose: Increase wrist motion; strengthen wrist muscles.

Precautions: If you have had wrist or elbow surgery, check with your doctor before doing this exercise. Stop if you feel any numbness or tingling.

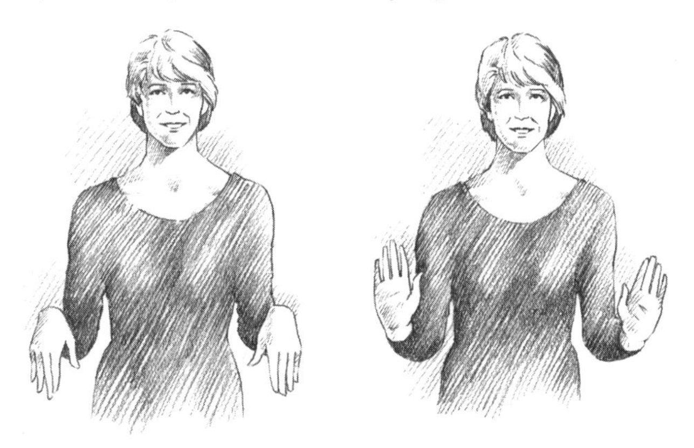

12. WRIST BEND

If sitting, rest hands and forearms on thighs, table, or arms of chair. If standing, bend your elbows and hold hands in front of you, palms down. Lift palms and fingers, keeping forearms flat. Hold three seconds. Relax.

FINGER EXERCISES

Purpose: Increase finger motion; increase ability to grip and hold objects.

Precautions: If the exercise increases finger pain, stop and consult with your doctor.

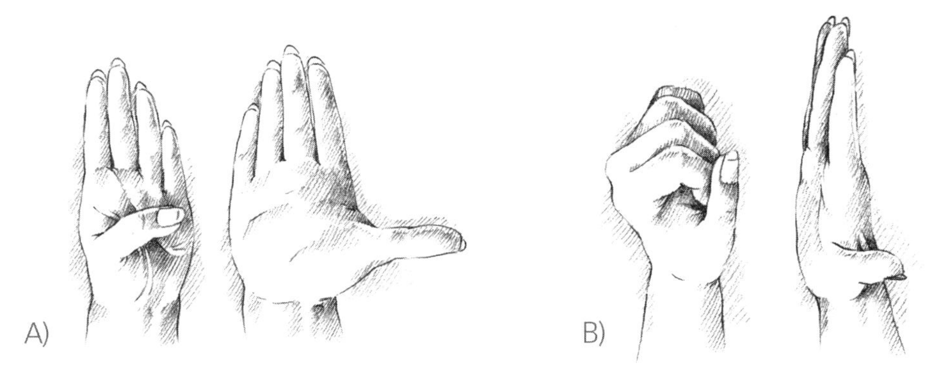

13. THUMB BEND AND FINGER CURL

(A) With hands open and fingers relaxed, reach thumb across your palm and try to touch the base of your little finger. Hold three seconds. Stretch thumb back out to the other side as far as possible. (B) Make a loose fist by curling all your fingers into your palm. Keep your thumb out. Hold for three seconds. Then stretch your fingers to straighten them.

TRUNK EXERCISES

Purpose: Increase trunk flexibility; stretch and strengthen back and abdominal muscles.

Precautions: If you have osteoporosis or have had back compression fracture, previous back surgery or a hip replacement, check with your doctor before doing these exercises. Do not bend your body forward or backward unless specifically told to do so. Move slowly and immediately stop any exercise that causes you back or neck pain.

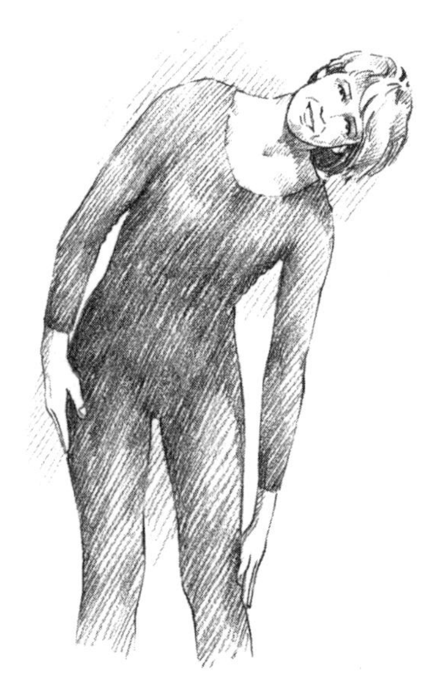

14. SIDE BENDS

While standing, keep weight evenly on both hips with knees slightly bent. Lean toward the right and reach your fingers toward the floor. Hold three seconds. Return to center and repeat exercise toward the left. Do not lean forward or backward while bending, and do not twist the torso.

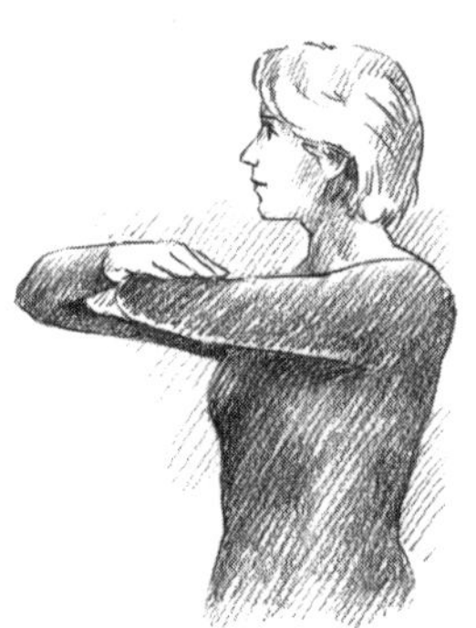

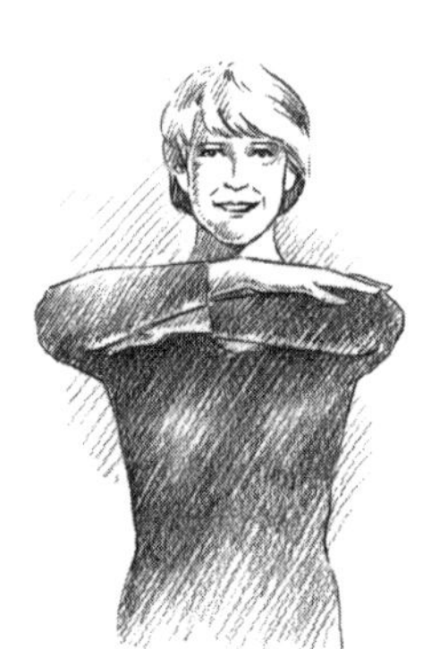

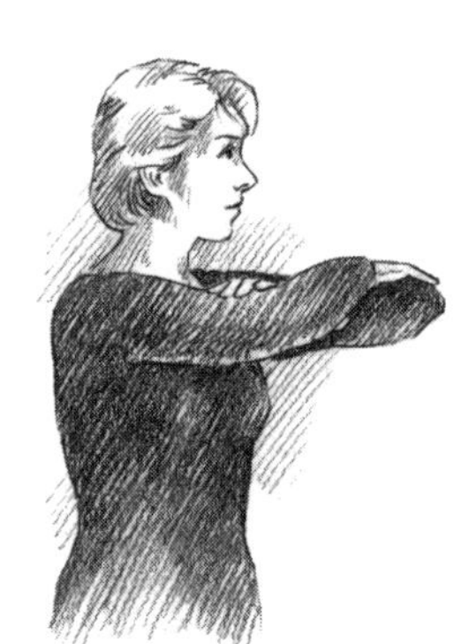

15. TRUNK TWIST

Place your hands on your hips, straight out to the side, crossed over your chest, or on opposite elbows. Twist your body around to look over your right shoulder. Hold three seconds. Return to the center and then twist to the left. Be sure you are twisting at the waist and not at your neck or hips. NOTE: Vary the exercise by holding a ball in front of or next to your body.

LOWER-BODY EXERCISES

Purpose: Increase lower-body strength; increase range of motion in hip, knee and ankle joints.

Precautions: Check with your surgeon before doing these exercises if you have had hip, knee, ankle, foot or toe surgery, or any lower-extremity joint replacement. Do not rotate the upper body unless specifically told to do so. When standing, bend your knees slightly to avoid "locking" your knee joints.

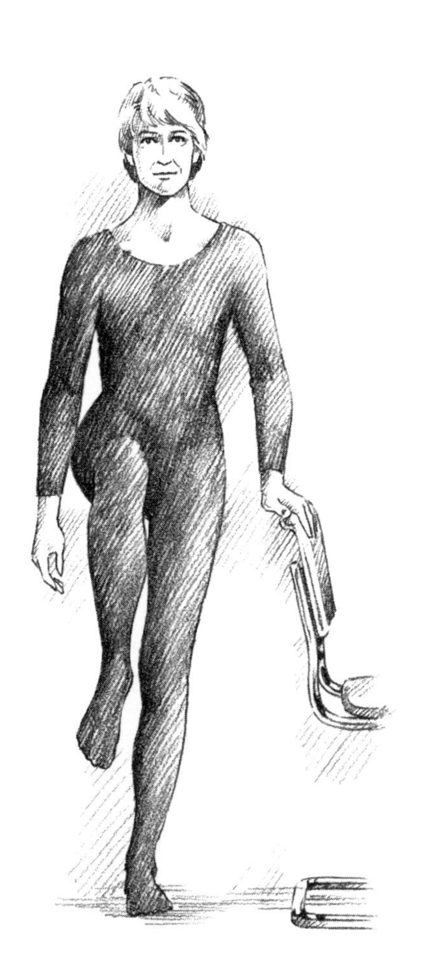

16. MARCH

Stand sideways to a chair and lightly grasp the back. If you feel unsteady, hold onto two chairs or face the back of the chair. Alternate lifting your legs up and down as if marching in place. Gradually try to lift knees higher and/or march faster.

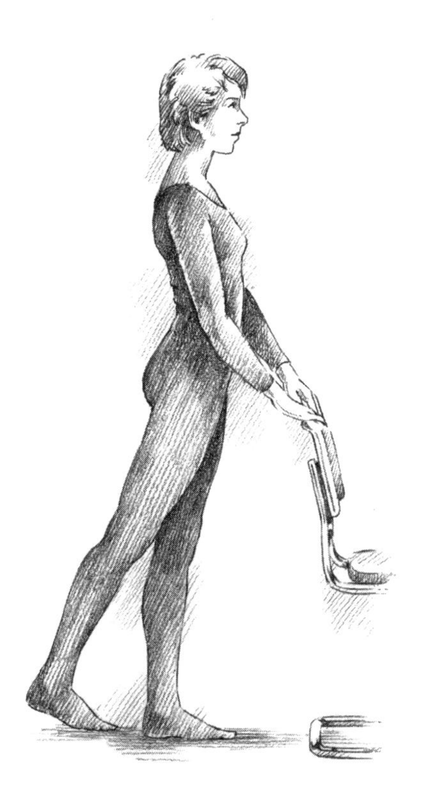

17. BACK KICK

Stand straight on one leg and lift the other leg behind you. Hold three seconds. Try to keep your leg straight as you move it backward. Motion should occur only in the hip (not the waist). Do not lean forward – keep your upper body straight. NOTE: You can add resistance by using a large rubber exercise band around ankles.

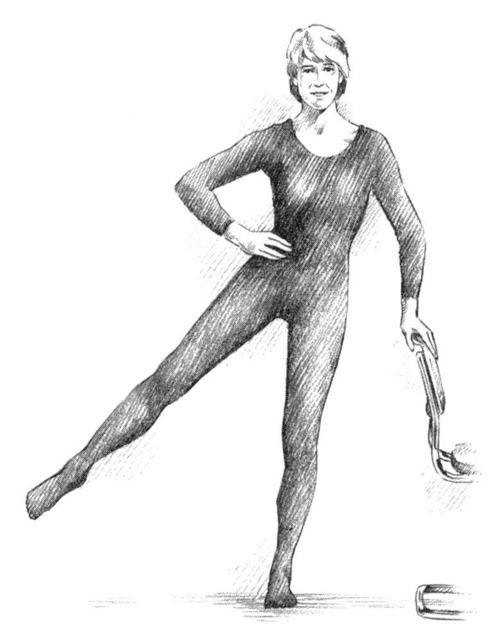

18. SIDE LEG KICK

Stand near a chair, holding it for support. Stand on one leg and lift the other leg out to the side. Hold three seconds and return your leg to the floor. Only move your leg at the top – don't lean toward the chair. Alternate legs.

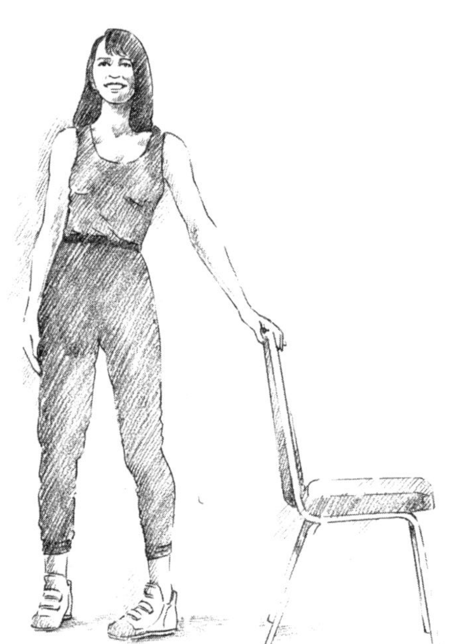

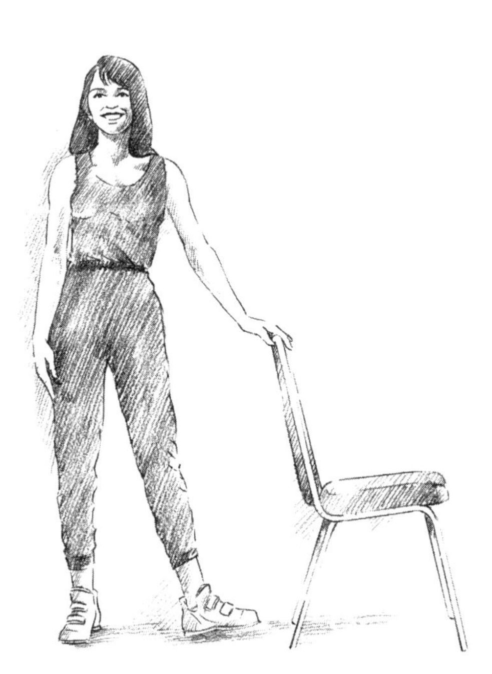

19. HIP TURNS

Stand with legs slightly apart, with your weight on one leg and the heel of your other foot lightly touching the floor. Rotate your whole leg from the hip so that toes and knee point in and then out. Don't rotate your body – keep chest and shoulders facing forward. NOTE: If you have difficulty putting weight on one leg, you can do this exercise by sitting at the edge of a chair with your legs extended straight in front and your heels resting on the floor.

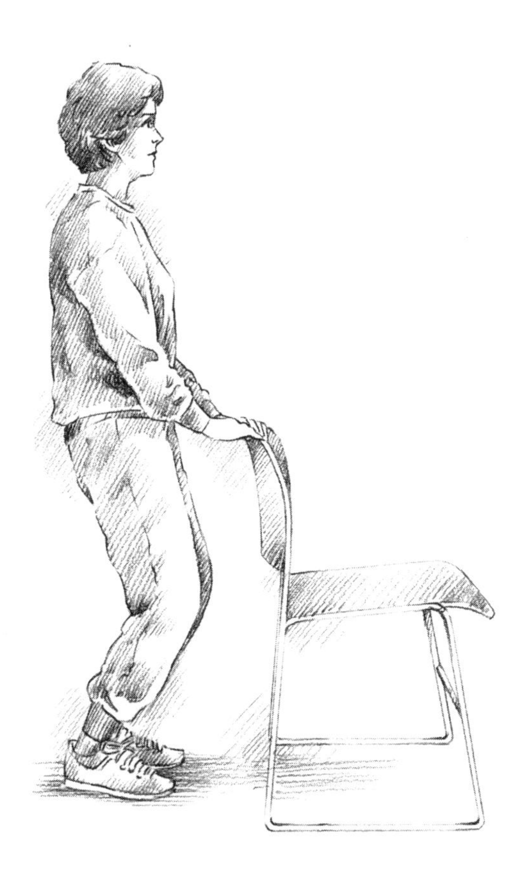

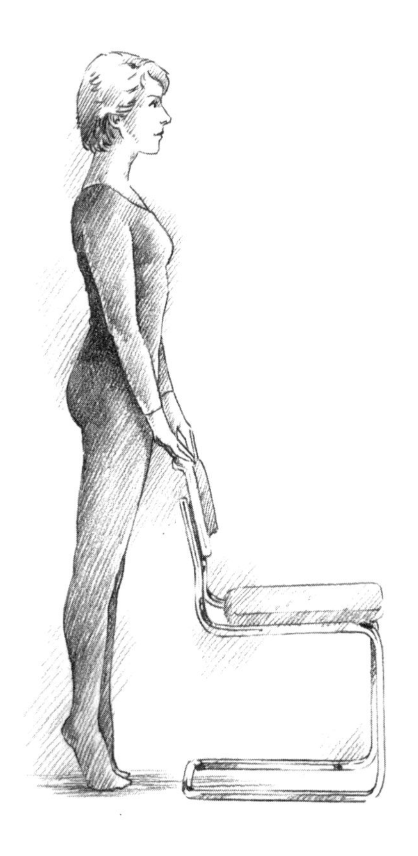

20. SKIER'S SQUAT (QUADRICEPS STRENGTHENER)

Stand behind a chair with your hands lightly resting on top of the chair for support. Keep your feet flat on the floor. Keeping your back straight, slowly bend your knees to lower your body a few inches. Hold for three to six seconds, then slowly return to an upright position.

21. TIPTOE

Face the back of a chair and rest your hands on it. Rise and stand on your toes. Hold three seconds, then return to the flat position. Try to keep your knees straight (but not locked). Now stand on your heels, raising your toes and front part of your foot off the ground. NOTE: You can do this exercise one foot at a time.

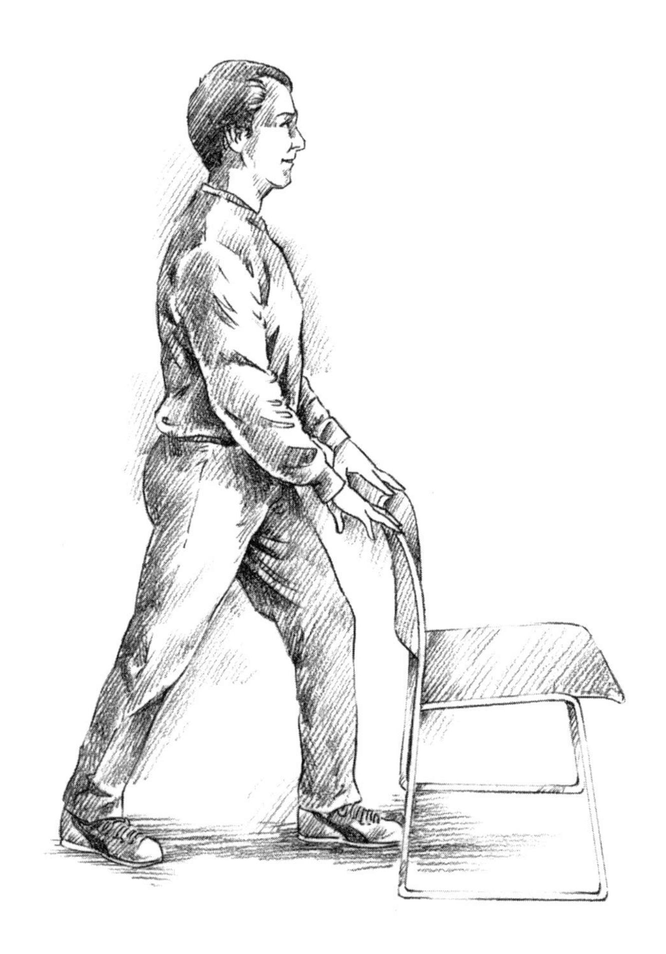

22. CALF STRETCH

Hold lightly to the back of a chair. Bend the knee of the leg you are not stretching so that it almost touches the chair. Put the leg to be stretched behind you, keeping both feet flat on the floor. Lean forward gently, keeping your back knee straight.

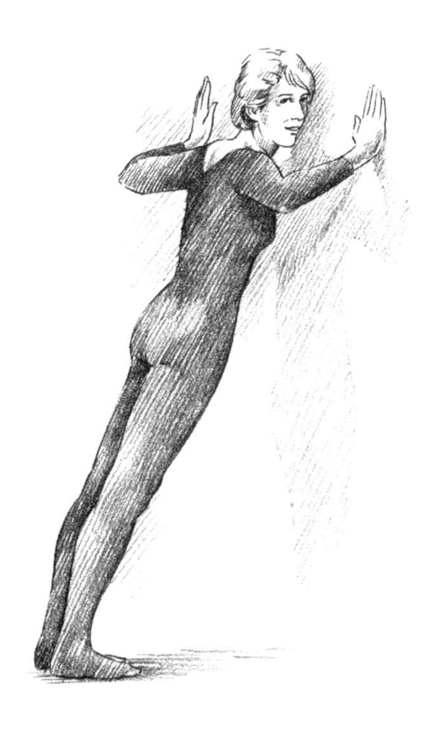

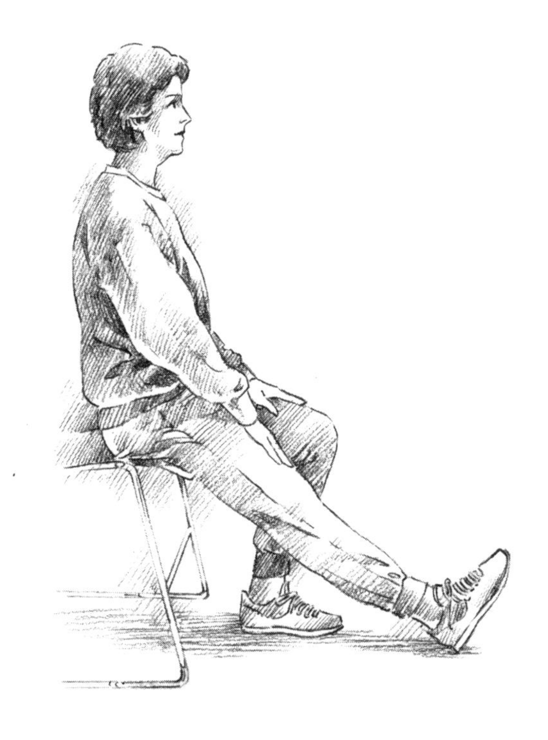

23. CHEST STRETCH

Stand about two to three feet away from a wall and place your hands or forearms on the wall at shoulder height. Lean forward, leading with your hips. Keep your knees straight and your head back. Hold this position for five to 10 seconds, then push back to starting position. To feel more stretch, place your hands farther apart.

24. THIGH FIRMER AND KNEE STRETCH

Sit on the edge of your chair or lie on your back with your legs stretched out in front and your heels resting on the floor. Tighten the muscle that runs across the front of the knee by pulling your toes toward your head. Push the back of the knee down toward the floor so you also feel a stretch at the back of your knee and ankle. For a greater stretch, put your heel on a footstool and lean forward as you pull your toes toward your head.

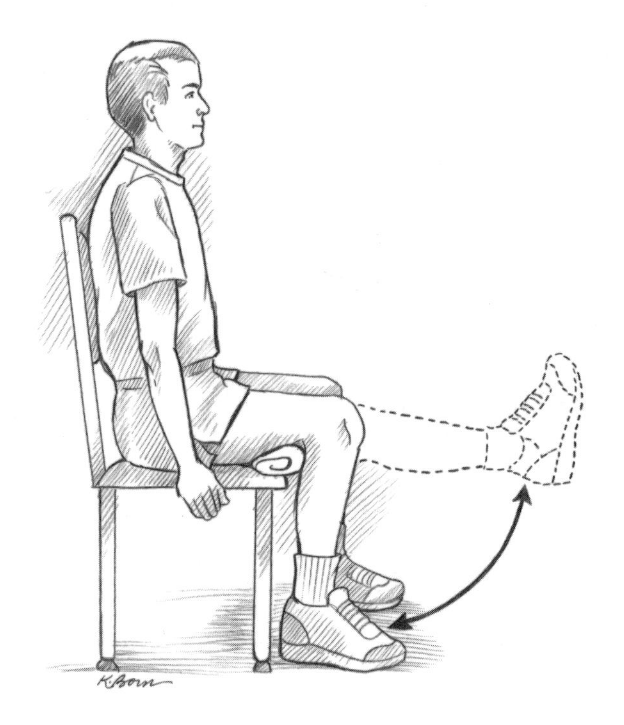

25. KNEE EXTENSION

Sit in a chair with your feet shoulder-width apart, knees directly above them. Put a towel under your knees for padding. With your hands on your thighs, raise your right leg to the count of three until your knee is straight (but not locked). Pause, then lower your leg to the count of three. Repeat on the left side.

(This exercise adapted from *Arthritis Today,* "Get Strong.")

Exercise Alternatives

We've suggested that in order to stay motivated to exercise, you choose activities that you like and that you change your routine periodically to keep things fresh. If you need a change, or if the activities covered don't appeal to you, feel free to investigate other options. Exercise has to be enjoyable to some degree if you're going to stick with it. You may be surprised at some of the exercise options that are available. Here are some additional activities you may want to try that might be so much fun you will forget they're exercise.

- Yoga. This ancient practice is considered a way of bringing the body, mind and spirit into harmony. In fact, the word "yoga" means "union." The practice of yoga can help strengthen muscles around affected joints and improve posture and balance to reduce stress on the joints. There are different schools of yoga, but all involve a series of postures called *asanas*. The practice of yoga often includes a meditation or relaxation component that promotes stress relief.

  Be sure to investigate a class carefully and talk with your doctor before you begin. Find out whether the yoga teacher is properly trained by checking with an organization such as the American Yoga Association. Some vigorous forms of yoga may not be appropriate for people with osteoarthritis.

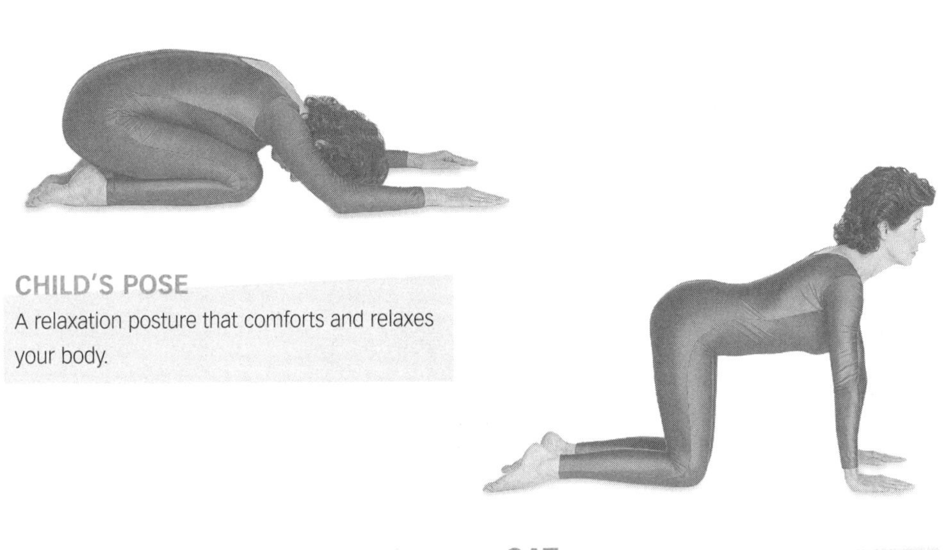

CHILD'S POSE
A relaxation posture that comforts and relaxes your body.

CAT
The cat pose stretches and strengthens the muscles of the low back.

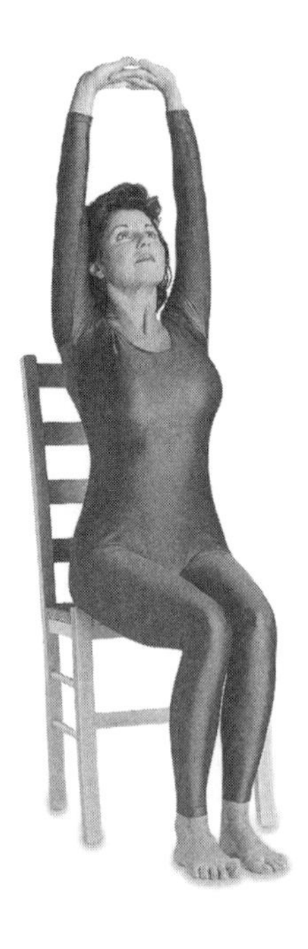

ARM STRETCH

This stretch opens up the rib cage and promotes shoulder range of motion.

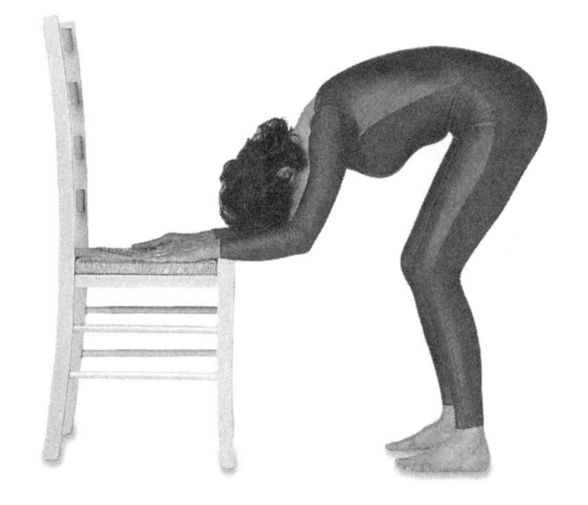

STANDING FORWARD BEND

Forward bending postures help keep the spine flexible. The pose is shown here modified with a chair.

• **Dancing.** Activities like ballroom dancing and other forms of dance can be effective and fun forms of exercise. They often incorporate vigorous movement that is considered to be aerobic. Like other forms of exercise, dance can improve flexibility and muscle tone. Dancing offers interaction with a partner or a group, which provides the added benefits of working out in a social setting. Music makes dance an especially enjoyable workout.

Before you begin, consult your doctor for any precautions or moves that you should avoid. Wear appropriate, stable shoes to prevent potential falls and injury. If you're a beginner, consider taking some classes so that you learn the steps and techniques properly.

• **Tai chi.** Tai chi is an ancient Chinese practice that involves gentle, fluid movements and meditation. This form of exercise often is recommended for people with musculoskeletal conditions like osteoarthritis because the soft movements are less stressful to the body and painful joints than other types of exercise. It is best to learn tai chi from a trained teacher. The soothing practice of tai chi helps strengthen muscles, improve balance and relieve stress.

Be sure to investigate the class and the teacher first. Check for an affiliation with a reputable health center.

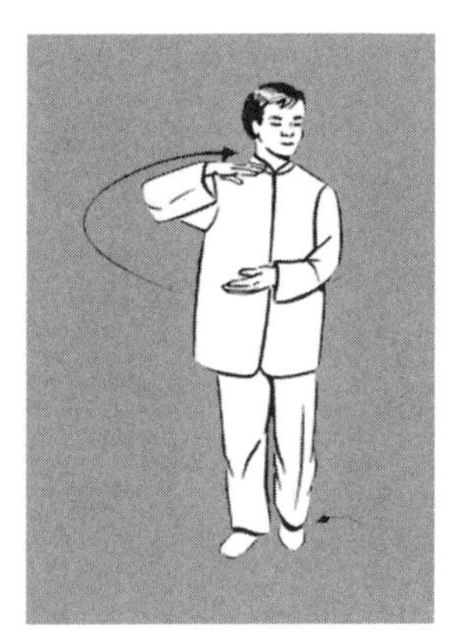
Part the Wild Horse's Mane *(Yema Fenzong)*

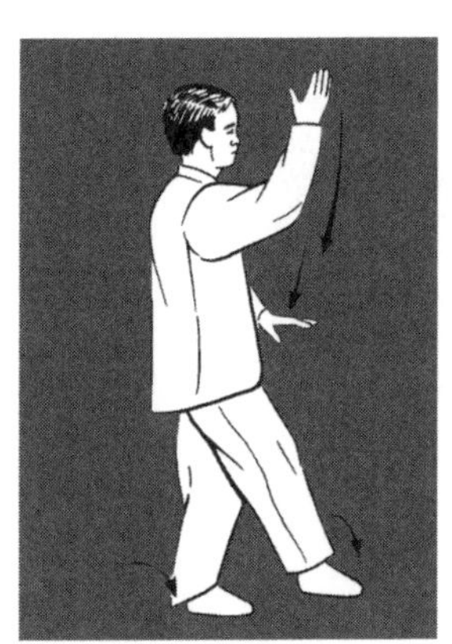
White Crane Spreads Its Wings *(Baihe Liangchi)*

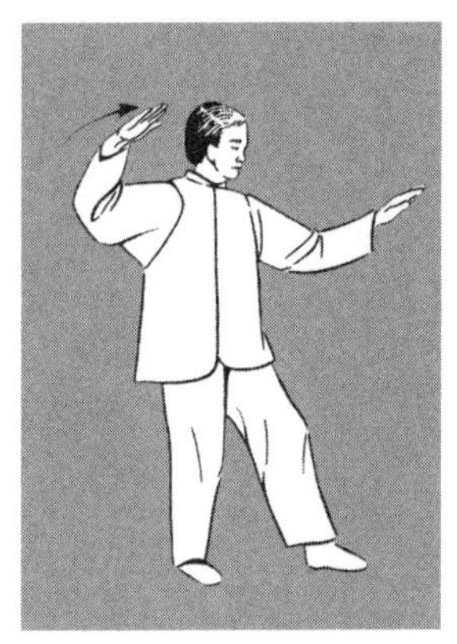
Reverse Reeling Forearm *(Daojuan Gong)*

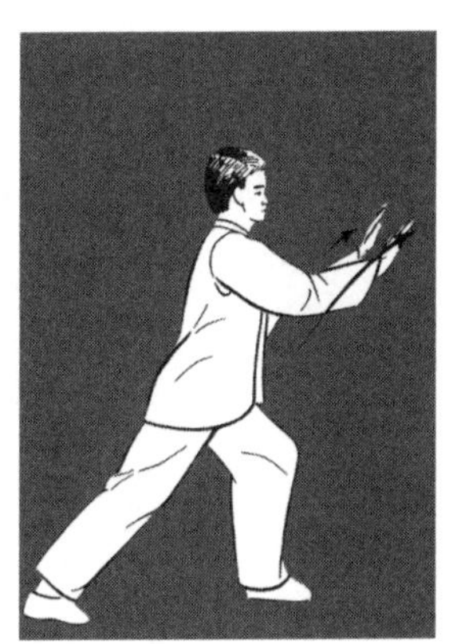
Grasp Sparrow's Tail *(Zuolan Quewel)*

Chapter 10

Diet Benefits: Maintaining Proper Weight for Joint Health

An important part of controlling osteoarthritis and preventing additional joint damage is maintaining a healthy body weight. As we've already seen in Chapter 1, being overweight can contribute to osteoarthritis by overloading your joints. The added stress may wear away protective cartilage more quickly, which can lead to joint damage and increased pain. Weight control and weight loss are a vital part of osteoarthritis treatment and prevention.

The Importance of Weight Control

In addition to easing the symptoms of osteoarthritis, maintaining a healthy weight has other significant health benefits. Research has shown that keeping extra pounds off can help reduce your risk for life-threatening diseases such as heart disease and cancer. It also gives you enough energy for your daily activities and helps you feel your best overall.

If you are already at an appropriate weight for your height, continue eating a healthy diet and exercising so that you don't gain extra pounds. If you are overweight, talk to your doctor about a safe and effective weight-loss plan to help minimize the effects of osteoarthritis.

Weight Loss Can Help...

- You feel better overall
- Take stress off your joints and reduce pain
- Prevent additional joint damage
- Reduce fatigue and increase energy

The Keys to Successful Weight Loss

New products or infomercials often promise "quick and easy" weight loss. But simply popping a pill can't make the pounds melt away. Although certain fad diets may help you take off pounds at first, deprivation tactics backfire. You eventually gain those pounds back – or more.

Talking with your doctor, a nurse or a nutritionist is the best way to start a successful weight-loss plan to make sure to get enough of the nutrients you need to stay healthy while you lose weight. Your doctor can guide you to a program that takes your needs and health background into account.

In addition to your doctor's recommendations, here are a few more strategies for a successful weight loss program.

- **Go gradually.** Researchers have found that people who make gradual lifestyle changes to lose weight are more successful than people who make drastic ones. If you slash calories too dramatically, you may not feel good and could set yourself up for failure. Most health professionals recommend that women eat no fewer than 1,200 calories per day, and men no fewer than 1,400 calories. Don't expect the pounds to come off immediately. Simply concentrate on making a habit of healthful eating and regular exercise.
- **Avoid absolutes.** Don't think of foods as "good" or "bad." If you think you can never have the so-called bad foods, you'll feel deprived, and you'll get discouraged if you slip up and eat them. Instead, consider high-fat, high-calorie foods as treats you can enjoy once in a while.
- **Add exercise.** In addition to eating well, be sure to get a good dose of exercise into your daily routine. This component of successful weight loss is discussed in more detail later in this chapter, but you should always be thinking about ways to get some activity into your day. If you don't have time for your 30-minute walk, cut it back to 10 minutes so you're still getting some exercise. Some exercise is always better than none at all.
- **Watch out for "fat-free."** Although the abundance of fat-free products may make you think that you can eat all those treats without the guilt, calories from fat aren't the only ones that can make you fat. All calories add up – and some fat-free products are still high-calorie enough to help you gain weight if you eat too much of them. Eat them in moderation.

What Is a Healthy Diet?

Nutrition and health experts offer several guidelines for eating a healthy diet that can help you maintain and even lose weight. You can use the guidelines to plan low-fat, low-calorie meals that include all the nutrients you need.

- **Eat a variety of foods.** A healthful diet typically includes selections from each of the five food groups that make up the Food Guide Pyramid: grains at least half of which are whole grains like whole-wheat flour products, oatmeal, brown rice; fruits; vegetables, including dark green and orange vegetables; and beans; low-fat dairy products; and low-fat meats and beans, especially fish. Beans, nuts and seeds are important sources of protein too. By choosing a range of foods from these different groups, instead of eating foods from just one or two groups, your body gets the 40 essential nutrients – i.e., nutrients your body cannot manufacture – it needs to function properly and stay healthy.

By eating a range of foods, you can usually keep your body supplied with the important nutrients. But talk with your doctor about how your medications may affect your body's intake of nutrients and whether a nutritional supplement would be helpful.

- **Consume fat and cholesterol in moderation.** Reducing the amount of fat and cholesterol in your diet may help reduce your risk for cardiovascular disease, maintain a proper weight or lose weight. Fat is a source of concentrated calories that can add extra pounds. Cholesterol, which is found in animal-based foods such as meat, can contribute to an increased chance of developing heart disease.

To lower the amount of fat and cholesterol in your diet, choose cuts of meat and dairy products that are lower in fat. Limit the amount of red meat and pork, oils, dressings, nuts and nut butters that you eat. Eat no more than three egg yolks per week.

- **Eat lots of fruits, vegetables and grains.** These foods are good sources of vitamins and minerals and are low in fat.

Guidelines for a Healthy Diet

Guidelines for a Healthy Diet
Eat a variety of foods.
Get the bulk of your fats from fish and plant sources such as nuts, seeds, and plant oils.
Eat plenty of fruits, vegetables and whole grains.
Cut back on sugar and salt.
If you drink alcohol, do so in moderation.
Drink eight glasses of water per day.

Foods such as beans, brown rice, whole grain breads and pasta are high in complex carbohydrates, which give your body energy. They are also high in fiber – the parts of plant foods that your body cannot digest – that not only helps keep you full, but also helps your body eliminate waste and prevents constipation.

Some types of fiber, such as oat bran, have been found to help lower cholesterol, and lower the risk of heart disease, some cancers, and diabetes. Research has found that dietary fiber also may be helpful in weight control by moderating insulin levels in the body. As with many other nutrients, it is best to get fiber from foods rather than from supplements.

- **Use sugar in moderation.** Sugary foods such as desserts and candy have now been booted from Food Guide Pyramid. Sugar adds calories that can contribute to weight gain, and it promotes tooth decay.

Although you may think that eating low-fat baked goods and desserts is fine, these products often contain lots of sugar

Making Meal Preparation Easier

Pain can reduce your appetite and make meal preparation more difficult. You may tend to avoid foods that take more time and effort to prepare. Here are a few ways that you can make meal preparation easier on your body so that it is easier to eat healthfully.

- Plan rest breaks during meal preparation.
- Use good posture to avoid pain during cooking tasks.
- Arrange your kitchen for convenience. Keep the tools you use most within easy reach.
- Buy healthy convenience foods such as sliced and chopped vegetables.
- Add fresh fruit and bread to a frozen dinner for a simple, satisfying meal.
- Use kitchen appliances and tools that save time and effort, such as electric can openers and microwave ovens.
- Share meals with friends or family members so you can split the cooking tasks and enjoy the company.

and may be high in calories. Moderating fat intake by choosing low-fat foods is important, but limiting calories is equally important. Something you'll accomplish by reducing the amount of sugar you consume. On food labels, look for the following words that indicate a product has added sugar: dextrose, sucrose, fructose, honey and dextrin.

- **Use salt (sodium) sparingly.** Most Americans consume far more sodium than they need. Sodium causes your body to retain water and, in salt-sensitive people can raise blood pressure. You can reduce sodium in your diet by resisting the temptation to shake salt on your food and using other seasonings, such as herbs, instead. Many packaged and prepared foods contain high levels of sodium, so check the label carefully. Look for low-sodium and no-salt-added versions of foods you eat frequently, especially canned vegetables and soups.
- **If you drink alcohol, do so in moderation.** Drinking excessive amounts of alcohol can have a number of negative effects on your body. It can weaken your bones, increasing the risk of osteoporosis, and add extra pounds.

Alcohol has the potential to interact with medications you may be taking for osteoarthritis. Stomach problems are more likely to occur if you drink alcohol and take aspirin or other NSAIDs. Drinking large amounts of alcohol and taking acetaminophen can damage the liver. Talk with your doctor or pharmacist about drinking any amount of alcohol if you take medications.

- **Drink eight glasses of water per day.** Your body needs water to maintain healthy tissues, to help flush waste and toxins, and to perform essential body functions. Drinking eight glasses each day gives your body the proper amount and keeps you from becoming dehydrated.

If you haven't been drinking that much water, it will take your body some time to adjust. At first, you may not want the water, and you may feel that you must run to the bathroom constantly. After a few days, your body should adjust.

Food Guide Pyramid

The Food Guide Pyramid, revised in 2005 by the U.S. Department of Agriculture and Health and Human Services, now emphasizes health as well as disease prevention. The pyramid is now sliced vertically: each slice represent one of the five food groups essential for a healthy diet. The groups – and the recommended amount to eat daily of each – are grains, especially whole grains, 6 oz.; vegetables,

THE USDA FOOD GUIDE PYRAMID

MyPyramid.gov
STEPS TO A HEALTHIER YOU

2.5 cups; fruits, 2 cups; dairy products, 3 cups; and lean proteins, 5.5 ounces. The USDA also recommends getting most of your fat from fish, nuts, and vegetable oils, like olive oil. It also notes that sugar adds "few, if any, nutrients" to a diet. Eating a variety of foods from the five groups each day will provide your body with the nutrients it needs to be healthy. Following the Food Guide Pyramid can help you balance your diet, lower your calories, and reduce sodium, sugar and saturated fat.

Reading Food Labels

Beginning in 1994, the U.S. government required that a new nutrition label appear on most foods. In addition to the ingredient lists already included on packages, this new label provides important nutrition information. It allows you to compare different foods by providing a standardized evaluation of the nutritional content, including fat, calories, cholesterol, sodium, fiber, protein, carbohydrates and vitamins.

The Food Labeling Act also set guidelines for health claims that could be made on food packaging. There are government standards for claims such as "low-fat," "fat-free" and "low-sodium." The foods must meet certain requirements before particular language can be used on the packaging. Following are some of the government definitions:

Light: 1/3 fewer calories or 1/2 the fat of the reference food. Sodium content of a low-calorie, low-fat food reduced by 50 percent.

Low: You can eat a large amount of this food without exceeding the daily value for the particular nutrient that is described as "low."

Fat-free: Contains less than 0.5 g fat per serving.

Fat-free Food: Naturally has no fat.

Lean: Less than 10 g of fat, less than 4 g of saturated fat, and less than 95 mg of cholesterol per serving and per 100 g.

Extra lean: Less than 5 g of fat, less than 2 g of saturated fat, and less than 95 mg of cholesterol per serving and per 100 g.

High: One serving of the food contains 20 percent or more of the daily value for the nutrient.

Good source: One serving of the food contains 10 to 19 percent of the daily value for the nutrient.

Food companies are also required to list the amount of trans fat – a hydrogenated fat common in processed foods like doughnuts and cookies – in the foods they produce. Trans fat, or hydrogenated fat, is associated with a higher risk of heart disease. Companies must now also identify any of the top eight allergens.

Controlling Portion Sizes

Many people are unsure of what constitutes a serving, or an appropriate portion size. If this is the case for you, you may be consuming more fat and calories than you realize, which could be adding extra pounds.

By being aware of portion sizes, you can control your intake of fat, calories and nutrients – and better control your weight. The following guidelines can help

Calorie Burning

The following chart can help you figure out how many calories you're burning during certain activities. The figures, from the American Dietetic Association, show the amount of calories burned per hour of activity.

Activity	120-lb person	150-lb person
Bicycling	178	210
Calisthenics	263	310
Dance exercise	289	340
Hiking	255	300
Jogging	552	650
Swimming (fast)	530	630
Swimming (slow)	272	320
Tennis	357	420
Walking	178	210

you visualize and understand appropriate serving sizes:

- 3 ounces of meat or fish: the size of a deck of cards or the palm of your hand
- 1 cup of vegetables: the size of your fist
- 1/2 cup of cooked pasta: an ice cream scoop full
- 1 1/2 ounces of cheese: a pair of dice or dominoes
- 1 teaspoon of butter or margarine: the tip of your thumb
- 1 cup of dry cereal: a large handful

Exercise for Weight Loss

In addition to eating a healthy diet, exercising regularly is an important component of a successful weight-control program. If you keep consuming the same amount of calories, you still can lose weight if you burn more calories through exercise and other physical activity.

Exercise is also key to your osteoarthritis treatment in order to keep your joints flexible and to maintain mobility. Along with strengthening and flexibility exercises that keep joints supported, aerobic exercise can help you control your weight. But don't think that you have to be an athlete to get the benefits. You simply need to pick activities you like and do them regularly. To boost your chances of success, choose a convenient activity that you enjoy and feel capable of doing on a regular basis. If the activity is too difficult, or too inconvenient, you're not likely to stick with it. For more details on creating your exercise program, see Chapter 9.

More Tips

You can increase your activity level and the calories you burn by adding bits of exercise throughout your day. Here are some suggestions:

- Stand up when you talk on the phone.
- Take the stairs instead of the elevator.
- Push the empty cart through the grocery store aisles first before you start shopping.
- Walk a lap through the mall before you browse in the stores.
- When you're watching TV, get up and walk around or fold laundry during the commercials.

PART FOUR

Assume Responsibility for What You Can Control

Chapter 11

Control the Hurt: Managing the Pain of Osteoarthritis

When your body is injured, the nerves of the damaged tissue trigger the release of chemicals. The chemicals relay messages to the brain, causing the unpleasant sensations that we call pain. And while you can't control the fact that you have pain, you can take steps to control it.

What Is Pain?

Pain has many causes as diverse as trauma and inflammation. Pain may be sharp or dull, chronic or acute, localized (felt in only one or two places) or generalized (felt throughout the body). In osteoarthritis, pain may be caused when the bones rub against each other because the cushioning cartilage tissue has worn away. Loose pieces of cartilage in the joint can also cause irritation and pain.

Individual responses to pain vary. What one person can barely feel, another can hardly tolerate. This is one reason your doctor relies on your reports of pain when examining you and when prescribing pain medications.

Pain can be measured on various scales, such as the visual analogue scale. To use the scale, you rate your pain on a scale of zero to 10 (or zero to 100), with zero indicating "no pain" and 10 (or 100) being the "worst pain imaginable." Keeping track of pain scores over time can help you and your doctor see how your disease is progressing and whether your pain medications are working.

The "Gate" Theory of Pain

Your nervous system plays an important role in how you experience pain. You may have heard reports about people with traumatic injuries who feel no pain immediately after an accident occurred. Somehow, the nervous system blocks the pain signals by using chemicals called *endorphins* that the body produces. Other situations can also trigger production of endorphins, such as the so-called "runner's high," which describes the euphoria experienced by runners in spite of their physical exertion.

Why is it that some pain signals get blocked? According to one theory, known as the gate-control theory of pain, when pain signals reach the nervous system, they stimulate a group of nerve cells that form a pain pool. When those cell reach a certain level of activity, a virtual gate opens, allowing the pain signals to proceed to higher pain centers in the brain.

Nondrug Strategies for Closing the Gate on Pain

Heat or cold treatments: These are usually applied directly to the site of pain. Heat may be more useful for chronic pain, cold packs for relief from acute pain.

Positive attitude and thoughts: Consciously switching to positive thoughts can distract your brain from feeling pain (see Chapter 13).

Exercise: Keeping your joints and muscles moving helps improve fitness and may decrease pain.

Relaxation techniques: You can train your muscles to relax and your thoughts to slow down by using these techniques, which include deep breathing, guided imagery and visualization.

Massage: When done properly, this method can relax your muscles and help you let go of tension.

Electrical stimulation: In this therapy called transcutaneous electrical nerve stimulation (TENS), electrodes stimulate large nerve fibers or cause the release of endorphins. TENS is usually prescribed by a doctor or physical therapist.

Topical lotions: These creams and rubs are applied to the skin over the painful muscle or joint. They may contain salicylates or capsaicin, compounds that decrease sensitivity to pain.

Acupuncture: A complementary or nontraditional therapy, acupuncture is the practice of inserting fine needles into the body along special points called meridians to relieve pain. (See the section on complementary and alternative therapies in Chapter 6.)

Sense of humor: Many studies have demonstrated that humor can increase the ability to handle pain.

The gate can also be closed by certain signals. Medications such as morphine and other narcotics block the pain signal, so the gate does not open.

Research has shown that, in addition to pain medication, nondrug methods can close the pain gate. Some or all of the strategies listed in the table below may help you deal with pain. Many of these strategies are discussed at greater length in this chapter or the chapters that follow.

Knowing what closes the pain gate can help you feel more in control. Use these strategies to create your own plan for dealing with pain. Be aware that, just as certain factors can close the pain gate, others can open it. Some of these, such as the pain from damaged cartilage or bone, may be beyond your control. But you can control other pain gate openers, at least in part. These include:

- overuse of pain medications
- overindulgence in alcohol
- extended periods of inactivity
- prolonged stress or anxiety
- too much physical activity/exertion
- obsessing about pain and negative thoughts

How to Manage Pain

The following is a list of some other steps that you may want to incorporate in your plan of action. Remember, not every technique will work for every person. Try a few of these, and if they don't work for you, try others.

- **Balance periods of activity with rest.** Just as doing too much can increase your pain, so can doing too little. Being inactive for long periods can make your joints stiffen, causing more pain when you try to move again. Try to balance your schedule so that you give your body appropriate amounts of moderate activity as well as time to rest and recover. To keep joints from becoming stiff, take time every day to move them through the range of motion that is possible.
- **Cut down on obligations.** Have a contingency plan for work obligations and family obligations. At work, try to arrange for coverage, work fewer hours per week, or bring work home. Discuss your plan with supervisors and co-workers ahead of time, and assure them of your commitment. At home, divide a few extra jobs among family members, and make sure everyone knows what they are expected to do to keep things running smoothly.
- **Communicate with your family and friends.** Let your family and friends know that you need more help. If someone volunteers to help you, give them a specific task. Otherwise, well-intentioned offers go

unused. There may be other sources of help available, such as members of your church or community volunteer organizations.

- **Practice relaxation or distraction techniques.** These techniques, discussed in Chapter 13, work best when you practice them regularly. Relaxation may not reduce your pain directly, but it can minimize stress, a factor shown to amplify pain.

There are many other techniques to use. When you find one that works for you, write it down and use it the next time you experience increased pain.

Managing Chronic Pain

Chronic pain – defined as pain that lasts longer than a few months – can be more challenging than acute pain. Handling the chronic pain and stiffness of osteoarthritis can lead to fatigue, discouragement or even depression. For some people with osteoarthritis, chronic pain becomes a constant companion. Learn to manage your chronic pain, so that you do not become its victim.

Some of the techniques for managing acute pain, such as relaxation, meditation and guided imagery, are helpful in reducing or minimizing chronic pain. The goal of the exercises is to train your brain and body to focus on positive and pleasing images, directing your attention away from pain. The effects of the techniques seem to build over time, so practicing them regularly is important for good results.

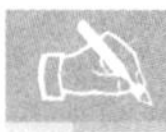

Personally Speaking STORIES FROM REAL PEOPLE

"I played the piano as a boy and later studied the accordion. I played classical and pop and other music. I'm now in my late 70s. Arthritis is with me. Finger pain. And I have tried all of the medications for joint relief. No help. NONE.

PLAY AND DO NOT STOP
– RAYMOND MINCHELLA, MESA, AZ

"How can one recapture the ease of fingering? Dexterity? The skill? I wonder: Can I make it to the next passage? Strike the next chord properly?

"I still try, I still play, and my mind tells me to go on. Don't stop. Play and do not stop. But the pain is there. Where is the secret? How can I feel pain-free?

"Mind over matter. I'll keep on trying. Or is it a dream, not to come true? I have hope. I won't give up."

Using Heat and Cold

Two of the simplest, least expensive and most effective methods of pain relief are heat and cold treatments.

Heat treatments, such as hot pads or warm baths, tend to work best for soothing stiff joints and tired muscles. Heat is especially good for getting your body limber and ready for exercise or activity. Cold is best for acute pain, numbing the painful area and decreasing inflammation and swelling.

There are many forms of heat and cold therapy. Experiment with some of the following ideas to find out which ones work best for you.

HEAT

- Take a long, warm shower when you awaken to ease morning stiffness.
- Try using a warm paraffin wax treatment system, available at many drugstores or beauty-supply stores.
- Soak in a warm bath or whirlpool.
- Buy a moist-heat pad from the drugstore, or make one at home by putting a wet washcloth in a freezer bag and heating it in the microwave for one minute. Wrap the hot pack in a towel and place it over the affected area for 15 to 20 minutes.
- To soothe stiff and painful joints in your hands, apply mineral oil to them, put on rubber dishwashing gloves, and place your hands in hot tap water for 5 to 10 minutes.
- Incorporate other warming elements into your daily routines, such as warming your clothes in the dryer before dressing, or using an electric blanket and turning it up for a few minutes before getting out of bed.

COLD

- Apply a bag of ice wrapped in a towel or a gel-filled cold pack from the drugstore to painful areas for about 10 minutes.
- Wrap a towel around a bag of frozen vegetables and place it on painful joints. This type of cold pack easily conforms to your body.

Safety Tips

When using heat and cold treatments, follow these steps to avoid injury, such as burns or ice burns:

- Use the heat or cold therapy for no more than 15 to 20 minutes at a time. Let your skin return to normal temperature before another application.
- Don't place the ice or hot pack directly on your skin. Always place a towel in between.
- Never use pain-relieving creams or gels with heat treatments.
- Don't sleep with an electric heating pad turned on.

WORKSHEET: My Pain-Management Plan

Use the following worksheet to record the strategies you plan to use for pain relief. That way you'll have a ready reference when you need it.

Medications: ______________________________

____

Schedule: ______________________________

____

____

Heat, cold, massage: ______________________________

____

Relaxation techniques: ______________________________

____

____

Exercises: ______________________________

____

____

Other techniques (distraction, humor, pleasant thoughts): ______________________________

____

____

Chapter 12

Avoiding Damage: Joint Protection Tips for Osteoarthritis

Another important way to manage pain is by taking steps whenever possible to avoid it. Remember that added pressure on already-weakened joints causes pain and possibly more damage to the joints.

What Is Joint Protection?

Joint protection refers to the ways you can make ordinary tasks easier on your joints so that you avoid damaging them. In addition to controlling osteoarthritis through weight loss, exercise and medications, you can make simple changes to daily activities that will reduce stress on your joints. Joint protection is another area where you can take control of osteoarthritis.

In addition to regular exercise for strengthening the areas around your painful joints, you can learn ways to use your joints carefully and reduce joint stress. Learning to listen to your body's signals when you need to rest is another way you can reduce pain, because preserving energy enhances your ability to deal with pain. Some of the most common techniques are described here, along with examples.

Good Body Mechanics

The term body mechanics refers to the way that you position and move your body to perform activities. Using good body mechanics means that you use techniques that put the least stress on your body for such tasks as standing, lifting and bending. The goal is to use your largest joints and muscles to perform the heaviest work so that smaller joints aren't overtaxed by tasks for which they weren't designed. By following the techniques of good body mechanics, you can protect and reduce pain in joints that are affected by osteoarthritis.

Posture

Poor posture can tire you and add to pain and stress on your joints. By using good posture, you put your body in the least stressful position and protect areas such as your neck, back, hips and knees.

- **Standing.** For proper standing posture, imagine a straight line that connects your ears, shoulders, hips, knees and heels. For good balance, keep your feet slightly apart or place one just in front of the other. Bend your knees slightly. Keep your stomach muscles tightened and your buttocks tucked under. Hold your chin in a comfortable position.
- **Sitting.** Keep your spine well supported while you are sitting. Keep your knees, hips and ankles at a 90-degree angle. Keep your shoulders back and your chin in a comfortable position.

Use Your Joints the Right Way

You can reduce pain and stress on your joints by following these tips to keep your body positioned the right way during everyday tasks.

- **Lifting and carrying.** Use the palms of both hands instead of just your fingers to carry items. When lifting, bend your knees and stand as you lift. Hold the item close to your body.
- **Climbing stairs.** Use railings for support and balance. Lead with your stronger leg when going up; lead with your weaker leg when going down.
- **Getting up from a chair.** Slide forward to the chair's edge and place your feet flat on the floor. Lean forward, then push down with your palms (not your fingers) on the arms or seat of the chair. Stand up by straightening your hips and knees.
- **Traveling.** Divide your items into two smaller, but equal loads, instead of one large bag. If possible, use a suitcase with wheels and an adjustable, pull-up handle.

Balancing Activity and Rest

Both physical activity and rest are important. The trick is in balancing them. Make moderation your motto, especially when your arthritis pain is worse.

Pace yourself by taking short breaks and alternating heavy and light activities during the day.

Set realistic goals for yourself. Make a "to do" list that isn't too long – and don't add to it.

Too much rest isn't good for your joints. Even on days when you're tired or stiff, try to do your exercises. You'll actually feel less stiff and have more energy if you do them.

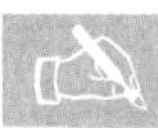

"Of course, I do not want to have arthritis. However, it has taught me patience in general, and the therapies I have explored have taught me many alternate ways of doing things.

"I have osteoarthritis in both hips; it is severe in my right joint and moderate in my left. This was discovered through X-rays my doctor ordered to account for leg pains I had been feeling for at least two years. My range of outward motion in each hip is quite limited – I find that I can no longer swing my leg over my bicycle's top bar. I cannot sit well in a chair or on a sofa, and car seats aren't any better. I walk kind of side to side. Sometimes, I cannot sleep well, especially on my right side (my favorite). Often, but not always, I cannot easily rise out of a chair and step forward. I cannot bend down easily to pick something off the floor.

ARTHRITIS IS A GREAT TEACHER
– FRED MARTINSON, KNOXVILLE, TN

"I must exercise every day. My wife and I began yoga. Yoga is the single best physical and mental therapy I have found – rising off the mat to the Standing Pose or bending over in the Hinge to get things off the floor have shown me new methods of moving. My posture is much better for standing, walking or sitting. I achieved a weight loss from 180 back down to 155 pounds by giving up all cookies, cakes and colas. This weight loss occurred fairly rapidly – in two to three months.

"My wife and I folk dance, and each week we do Scandinavian and international styles with two different groups. Although my range of motion is affected, the exercise, music and friends help physical problems disappear.

"One of my biggest helps is my wife, Nancy. She encourages me, and we do a number of things together. We belong to an interfaith meditation group, and those friends, that practice, and some reading on the subject are an immense help. That dimension of my life, my spiritual practice, is one of the most important things in my life.

"I keep rough journals noting when I add supplements, for example, and I jot down any changes. I attend the local arthritis support group and find it helpful. Our local chapter of the Arthritis Foundation is very helpful with activities, books, videos and the like.

"One of the scariest things I have done in coping with my arthritis is to go see a surgeon who performs hip replacements; my doctor had said I might need that. I might, but for the time being, I have found that the exercises I do, the supplements I take, plus the spiritual practice I have are helping me maintain the life I enjoy. I feel very lucky."

Schedule your breaks – and take them. Don't wait for physical signals of pain before you rest.

Get Organized

We would all like to be more organized and efficient in our daily lives. Organization is especially helpful if you have osteoarthritis, because the energy you save in daily activities will allow you to do more of the things you enjoy. Here are simple ways you can get things in order.

- If you work, keep all equipment and tools within easy reach and at a comfortable level. Use a lazy Susan or storage bins to keep supplies handy.
- Streamline cleaning chores by using an all-in-one cleaning product or one that reduces scrubbing. Don't try to clean everything in one day – rotate the tasks over the course of the week.
- When doing household repairs like fixing a sink, gather all the necessary tools or use a toolbox, so you don't have to continually get up and down. Ask the clerk at your hardware store for tools with special grips that are easier to handle.
- When cooking, put all necessary tools and ingredients on the counter before you start; that will minimize trips to the pantry and refrigerator. Use convenience foods – such as precooked, cubed chicken– to save energy, and wear and tear on joints.
- Organize your errands. If your bank is next door to the dry cleaner, make one trip instead of two.

Self-Help Devices

When you're tired, stiff or in a hurry, self-help devices can make tasks easier on your joints and you more efficient. The products, which range from the simple to the elaborate, help keep joints in the best position for function, provide leverage, and extend your range of motion. You can find simple devices such as jar openers, reachers and easy-grip utensils in many hardware stores, medical supply stores and even discount stores. In fact, design that increases ease is a growing trend; even products marketed to the general public are incorporating more of these design features.

- Zipper pulls and buttoning aids can help you fasten clothing more easily. Or you can opt to wear clothing with Velcro fasteners. A long-handled shoehorn extends your reach and prevents bending.
- In the kitchen, appliances such as electric can openers and food processors make work easier. Reachers can be used to retrieve items stored high or low. Built-up handles and grips make utensils easier to grasp and put less stress on your finger joints.

Finding Self-Help Devices

The companies listed below offer ergonomic equipment for the office and the home. This list is by no means complete, but it may give you a good place to begin searching for useful products. Consult a physical or occupational therapist, or speak to your doctor, to find more sources of self-help or assistive devices.

You can request catalogs from these companies and order items on your own, or you can order products through a physical or occupational therapist.

DAILY LIVING EQUIPMENT

Aids For Arthritis, Inc.
35 Wakefield Drive
Medford, NJ 08055
800-654-0707
www.aidsforarthritis.com

Assistive Devices, Inc. (ADI)
4000 Brandi Court
Austin, TX 78759-8109
800-856-0889
512-346-0889
www.assisteddevicesinc.com

Concepts ADL
10804 Mark Twain Road
West Frankfort, IL 62896
800-626-3153
www.adlrehab.com

Kinsman Enterprises
10804 Mark Twain Road
West Frankfort, IL 62896-4105
618-932-3838
www.kinsmanenterprises.com
This company manufactures products to help people do everyday tasks more easily. Contact the company for information about where to buy the products.

North Coast Medical
Consumer Products Division
18305 Sutter Blvd.
Morgan Hill, CA 95037
800-235-7054
www.ncmedical.com
NCM offers catalogs featuring products to help with everyday living and workplace needs.

Patterson Medical Company
P.O. Box 5071
Bolingbrook, IL 60440
800-558-8633
www.sammonspreston.com

Sears Health and Wellness Catalog
7700 Brush Hill Road
Burr Ridge, IL 60527
800-326-1750
www.searshealthandwellness.com

ERGONOMIC OFFICE EQUIPMENT

ErgoDirect
19 Newport Ave.
Selden, NY 11784
866-374-6347
www.ergodirect.net

Ergo Source
P.O. Box 695
Wayzata, MN 55391
www.ergosource.com
To receive their information, leave a message requesting company literature. Products include office accessories, forearm supports, foot rests and adjustable work surfaces.

Infogrip
1794 East Main Street
Ventura, CA 93001
805-652-0770
800-397-0921
info@infogrip.com
www.infogrip.com

- In the bathroom, tub bars and handrails provide additional stability and security when you are getting into and out of the bathtub or shower. Faucet levers or tap turners are available if your grip is weak. An elevated toilet seat can make it easier to sit down on and get up from the toilet.
- Many devices and modifications are available for a work environment, from adjustable-height chairs and work surfaces to telephones with large push buttons and ergonomic computer keyboards. If you need modifications at work, see an occupational therapist. He or she can help you make changes and find the devices you need.
- You can still enjoy leisure activities by using assistive devices such as kneelers and lightweight hoses for gardening, "no-hands" frames for quilting or embroidering, and card holders and shufflers for playing cards.

PART FIVE

Master Emotional Challenges

Chapter 13

Learning To Relax: Ways to Manage Stress Effectively

Dealing with stress is a daily challenge for everyone, not just those with chronic illnesses like osteoarthritis. By learning to control your stress, you can reduce your pain, feel healthier and manage your condition more effectively.

What Is Stress?

Stress refers to how the body reacts – physically and mentally – to situations that are exciting, dangerous or annoying. Too much stress can worsen pain and other symptoms of osteoarthritis.

Yet stress is a normal part of life. A move to a different town, a new job, a divorce, or the death of someone close to you – all those can be stressful. But stressful events aren't always negative ones. Weddings, births and vacations are happy occasions that can also bring on stress.

People with osteoarthritis go through the same stressful periods as everyone else. Having a chronic health condition can add a new set of challenges and daily adjustments. You may have to rely on family members and health-care professionals more than in the past. You may have to alter your lifestyle or give up favorite activities because of limited abilities. None of these changes is easy – and all of them can be upsetting. But you don't have to let them get you down. You can learn to understand and manage your stress so the adjustments will be easier to handle.

Positive Stress vs. Negative Stress

Stress is supposed to be a temporary response, a sort of emergency setting that revs our engines and shifts us into high gear, enabling us to cope with difficult situations. But if you get stuck on that setting, stress becomes unhealthy. Here are some differences between healthy and unhealthy stress reactions:

Healthy stress is followed by relaxation. Your resources balance out your demands. After you've dealt with the situation, your body returns to its pre-stressed state – heartbeat and breathing slow, blood pressure goes down, and muscles relax. Your physical and emotional energies recharge, so that you can meet the next challenge.

Unhealthy stress occurs when your perceived demands exceed your perceived resources. You stay geared up. Your body is still in a stressed state – heart racing, blood pressure up, muscles tight, palms sweaty, stomach knotted. Because you aren't relaxing, your body and mind are unable to recover energy and balance, so the next challenge is difficult to meet. With each challenge, your physical and emotional resources become more exhausted. The stress has become chronic. Chronic stress can cause many negative effects on your body and mind. (See Effects of Chronic Stress on opposite page.)

How Your Body Reacts to Stress

When you feel stressed, your body becomes tense. This muscle tension can increase pain, making you feel helpless and frustrated because the added pain may limit your abilities. This, in turn, can depress you. Stress, depression, and limited

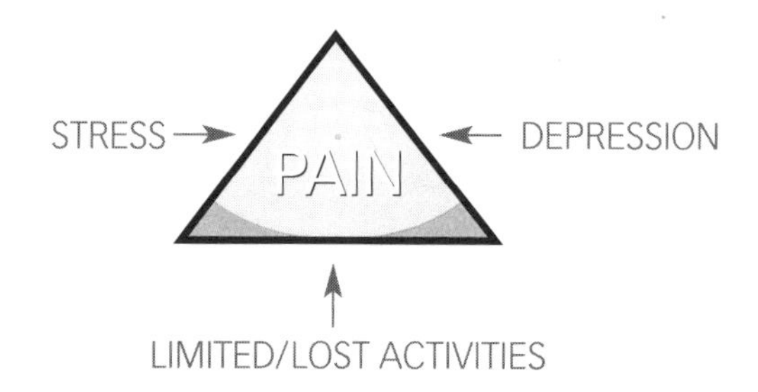

Stress, depression, and limited/lost activities can all contribute to pain.

and lost abilities can all contribute to pain, which then perpetuates a cycle of stress, pain, limited and lost abilities, and depression. If you understand how your body reacts physically and emotionally to stress and learn how to manage stress, you can help break that destructive cycle.

Physical Changes

Some of your body's reactions to stress are easy to predict. At stressful times, the body releases epinephrine chemicals into your bloodstream. This sets in motion a series of physical changes called the fight-or-flight response. Your heart beats faster as your breathing rate increases. Blood pressure rises, and your muscles feel tense.

The physical changes give you added strength and energy. They prepare your body for dealing with stressful events, such as giving a speech before a large audience. When stress is handled in a positive way, the body restores itself and repairs any damage caused by the stress.

At times, you may feel unable to deal with stress in a positive way. As a result, stress-related tension builds up, and with no outlet, takes its toll on your body. This toll can take many forms – headaches, upset stomach or worsened osteoarthritis symptoms. Research shows that stress affects the body's immune system, leading to illness, fatigue or other physical problems. And according to a review of nearly 300 studies on stress and health, those who are older or already sick, are more vulnerable to stress-related immune changes.

Emotional Changes

Your mind's reaction to stress is harder to predict than your physical reaction. Emotional reactions vary, depending on the situation and the person. They may include feelings of anger, fear, anxiety, helplessness, loss of control, annoyance or frustration. A small amount of stress can actually help people perform their best – during an exam, a stage performance or athletic event, for example. But under too much stress, people may become accident-prone, commit errors and perform clumsily.

Each person responds to stress differently. You may like to be busy, or you may prefer a slow pace with less activity.

Effects of Chronic Stress

Effects of Chronic Stress
Headaches
Stomach distress, ulcers
High blood pressure
Muscle tension, back pain and other types of pain
Chronic fatigue
Restlessness, irritability, frustration
Decreased zest for life, worry, fear, depression
Difficulty making decisions, forgetfulness
Increased use of alcohol, cigarettes or drugs
Eating and sleeping problems
Disease flares
Poorer immune function

What you find relaxing may be stressful to someone else.

Managing Stress

The key to managing stress is to make it work for you instead of against you. Consider the following steps to a complete program for managing your stress.

- Recognize your body's stress signals.
- Identify what causes your stress.
- Change what you can to reduce stress.
- Manage or accept what you can't change.
- Adopt a lifestyle that builds resistance to stress.

Diagnosing Your Stress Symptoms

Just as perception of stress is a personal matter, the same is true for how stress affects us physically and emotionally. One person's stress is manifested by headaches and tight shoulder muscles. Another person seldom gets headaches but gets an upset stomach.

Stress symptoms often are obvious, but not always. For example, a stress headache may begin as a slightly aching neck that you ignore (it doesn't really hurt, you tell yourself) until it turns into a pounding headache. Or you may assume that your upset stomach was caused by something you ate – until you notice the same thing happens every time you confront a stressful situation. By listening to your body, you can learn how stress affects you. (See the sample diary below.)

Sample Stress Diary

DATE	CAUSE OF STRESS	TIME	PHYSICAL SYMPTOMS	EMOTIONAL SYMPTOMS
4/18	getting kids off to school	7 a.m.	fast heartbeat, tightness of neck	feel rushed, disorganized
4/18	stuck in traffic	8:30 a.m.	headache, heart beating faster, legs aching	frustrated, angry at being late
4/18	meeting presentation	10 a.m.	fast heartbeat, dry throat, clammy palms	anxious, nervous

Identifying the Causes of Your Stress

What causes you the most worry and concern? What situations leave you anxious, nervous or afraid? Once you recognize the stressful aspects of your life, you can decide how to change them or adapt to them.

Keeping a Stress Diary

Record the events in your life that cause stress, as well as any physical or emotional symptoms that result. After one week, look for patterns in symptoms, determine what causes them and make life adjustments.

DATE	CAUSE OF STRESS	TIME	PHYSICAL SYMPTOMS	EMOTIONAL SYMPTOMS

Listening To Your Body

Be aware of:

1. Headaches
2. Stomach upset
3. Emotional reactions
4. Sleeping problems
5. Other signs

Some Warning Symptoms

1. Tight shoulder, arm or neck muscles
   Hunched shoulders
   Clenched teeth
2. Stomach knot or butterflies
   Stomach ache
   Appetite loss
   Diarrhea or constipation
3. Anxiety
   Moodiness
   Anger
   Hopelessness
   Low self-esteem
   Poor concentration
   Depression
4. Trouble falling asleep
   Waking up early, being unable to fall asleep again
   Oversleeping, sleeping too much
   Disturbing dreams
5. Chronic fatigue
   Cold, clammy hands
   Heart pounding
   Chest feels tight or heavy
   Dry mouth

Changing and Managing the Causes of Stress

Once you've identified the causes of your stress, determine which stressful situations can be changed and which cannot. Take action to change what you can control. The following strategies may help.

- Set goals and develop a plan of action for reaching them. Delegate responsibilities to friends or family members. Try to be flexible about timelines you set for a goal so you can accommodate osteoarthritis.
- List your priorities. What needs to be done immediately? What can be done later? What can be eliminated? You may need to buy groceries today so you have food for dinner, but maybe something else like washing clothes can wait until tomorrow.
- Reduce the hassles in your day. If rush-hour commuting bothers you, map out a new way to work – a longer one, if necessary – to avoid high-traffic areas. Has anyone really noticed or rewarded the times you've stayed late at work compared with the effects this overtime has had on your health? The company will survive if you scale back your hours. If certain people or places annoy you, avoid them. If you have to put up with them, decide at the outset that you won't allow them to get on your nerves.

- Aim to have more uplifting than aggravating activities in your life. Make a list of each and compare them. Think about ways you can increase the uplifting and decrease the frustrating ones.
- When making a decision about whether or not to take on a task, ask yourself, "Am I taking care of my needs?" It's easy to become caught up in caring for others at the expense of your own health. Take time to pamper yourself and do things you enjoy rather than sacrifice your needs all the time.
- Plan ahead for special events so you can enjoy them rather than collapse from stress. Shop early or year-round for holiday and birthday gifts so you won't be caught in a last-minute crush. Buy many cards at once – for birthdays, weddings, new babies and anniversaries – so you'll have them on hand. If you're entertaining, make realistic decisions about foods you can cook easily and buy the rest. Or make it a potluck bash.
- Learn to say *no* without feeling guilty. It's fine to bow out of activities when you don't feel up to them. Turning down extra duties can reduce your stress.
- Seek solutions that benefit both sides in a conflict. If you want to go for a walk and your spouse has chores to do, help finish the work and go walking together.

Reality Check

Learn to put stressful situations in perspective by asking these questions:

- Does this situation reflect a threat by signaling harm or a challenge by signaling an opportunity?
- Are there other ways to look at this situation?
- What exactly is at stake?
- What is the worst that can happen?
- What am I afraid will occur?
- What evidence do I have that this will happen?
- Is there evidence that contradicts this conclusion?
- What coping resources are available?

If You Can't Change the Situation, Change Your Outlook

You can only change yourself, not other people. Some situations can't be changed, but your point of view can. Try to roll with the punches. Being flexible helps you keep a positive attitude despite hardships. Here are some ways to help you change your outlook.

ACTIVITY: Deep Breathing

Deep breathing is a basic technique that applies to almost all relaxation exercises. This simple technique is the key to mastering the art of unwinding. Here are the steps:

1. Get as comfortable as you can. Loosen any tight clothing or jewelry, uncross your legs and arms. Close your eyes.

2. Place your hands firmly but comfortably on your stomach. This will help you feel when you are breathing properly. When you breathe correctly, your stomach expands as you breathe in and contracts when you breathe out. (Many people do the opposite – they tighten their stomachs when they breathe in and relax their stomachs when they breathe out. If you do, take a minute to reverse.)

3. Inhale slowly and deeply through your nose to a count of three. Do you feel your stomach push against your hands? Let it expand as much as possible as you fill your lungs with air.

4. When your lungs are full, purse your lips as if you were going to whistle, and exhale slowly through your mouth for a count of six. Pursing your lips allows you to control how slowly or quickly you exhale. Do you feel your stomach shrink away from your hands?

5. When your lungs are empty, close your mouth and begin the inhale/exhale cycle again.

6. Repeat the inhale/exhale cycle three or four times at each session.

7. Whenever you're ready, slowly open your eyes and stretch.

Tip: Breathing deeply can make you feel light-headed or dizzy – especially when you are tired or hungry. It's a good idea at first to practice deep breathing while you are sitting or lying down. Once you get the hang of it, deep breathing can be used anytime, anywhere.

- **Think positively.** Ask yourself if there is any hidden benefit to the stressful situation, and make the most of it. Getting fired or laid off from a job could lead to a spiral of depression, debts and debilitating pain. Or it could be the opportunity you've been looking for to change your work situation for the better.
- **Do a reality check.** Try to evaluate the situation's real importance. Your daughter didn't call this week. Does it mean she's ignoring you, or that her own schedule was difficult to manage? And will your world collapse because she didn't call?
- **Develop and use support systems.** Share your thoughts with family, friends, clergy or others who are good listeners and can help you see the problems in a constructive way. However, don't whine to others about every detail of your discomfort. You may alienate your support structure and isolate yourself from the help you need, and you may be reinforcing a bad habit of focusing on your pain.
- **Refocus your attention.** Thinking about something or someone else besides yourself can help you relax and distract you from pain.
- **Develop "safety valves."** Release stress by working it out with exercise or by writing in a journal.

Relaxation Tips

- Pick a quiet place and time of day when you won't be disturbed for at least 15 minutes.
- Make yourself as comfortable as possible before beginning. Loosen any tight clothing and uncross your legs, ankles and arms. Sit in a comfortable chair or lie down.
- Try to relax daily or at least four times a week.
- Don't expect immediate results. It may be several weeks before you reap benefits from some techniques.
- Relaxation should be enjoyable. If these techniques are unpleasant or make you more nervous and anxious, stop. You may manage your stress better with other techniques.

- **Have fun.** Schedule time for play and join activities that make you laugh. See Chapter 8 for more about the healing qualities of humor.

Relaxing To Reduce the Effects of Stress

Learning how to relax is one of the most important ways you can cope with stress. Relaxation is more than just sitting back and being quiet. It is an active process, requiring practice, to calm your body and mind. Once you know how, relaxing becomes second nature. As you learn new methods, keep these principles in mind.

- Stress has many causes, which means there are many solutions. The better you understand what causes your stress, the more successfully you can manage it.
- Not all relaxation techniques will work for everyone. Whatever works for you is what's important. Try different methods. You may learn that some techniques work well for certain situations, while others

ACTIVITY: Relaxation To Control Pain

Preparation: First, take time to make sure that you are in a comfortable position. Check from head to toe to determine whether your whole body is supported. Adjust any parts that feel uncomfortable. Try not to have legs or arms crossed, but above all, do what is comfortable for you.

Now, close your eyes. Become aware of your breathing. Feel the movement of your body as you breathe in and out. Breathe in slowly and exhale. On your next breath, focus on an image of breathing in good, clean air and exhaling all your tensions with your breath out. Slow your breathing and focus on releasing tension each time you breathe out.

Middle Part:

Option 1: "Pain Drain" Feel within your body, and note where you experience pain or tension. Imagine that the pain or tension is turning into a liquid substance. The heavy liquid flows down through your body and out through your fingers and toes. Allow the pain to drain from your body in a steady flow. Now, imagine that a gentle rain flows down over your head and further dissolves the pain into a liquid that drains away. Enjoy the sense of comfort and well-being that follows.

Option 2: "Disappearing Pain" Notice any tension or pain that you are experiencing. Imagine that the pain takes the form of an object or several objects. It can be fruit, pebbles, crystals or anything that comes to mind. Pick up each piece of pain, one at a time, and place it into a magic box.

As you drop each piece into the box, it dissolves into nothingness. Again survey within your body to see if any pieces remain and remove them. Imagine that your body is work better at other times.

- Learning these new skills will take time. Practice new techniques for at least two weeks before you decide if they work well for you.

If you need help learning how to relax, see a mental health professional or contact your local Arthritis Foundation chapter. A few common techniques for relaxing are described below, as well as several relaxation activities. Contact your local Arthritis Foundation chapter for information on audiocassettes you can purchase to accompany these activities.

lighter, and allow yourself to experience a feeling of comfort and well-being. Enjoy the feeling of tranquility and repose.

Option 3: "Healing Potion" Imagine you are in a drugstore stocked with bottles and jars of exotic potions. Each potion has a special magical quality. Some are pure, white light, others are lotions, balms and creams, and yet others contain healing vibrations. As you survey the potions, choose one that appeals to you. It may even have your name on the container. Open the container and cover your body with that magical potion. As you apply it, let any pain or tension melt away, leaving you with a feeling of comfort and well-being. Imagine that you place the container in a special spot and that it continually renews its contents for future use.

Option 4: "Leaving Pain Behind" Imagine that you are dreaming and that you are leaving your body behind. As you leave, notice that you have also left your tension and pain behind. Pick a special spot to visit, one that brings pleasure and a feeling of well-being. Notice how your dream-like body feels as you visit this special place. Linger here for a while and when you feel ready, return to your body. When you open your eyes, retain the freedom from tension and pain, and continue to experience a sense of comfort and well-being.

End Part:

Whenever you are ready, slowly stretch and open your eyes.

Adapted from The ROM Dance, a range-of-motion and relaxation program by Diane Harlowe and Patricia Yu, 1992. Materials available from Tai Chi Health with Tricia Yu, 408 S. Baldwin St., Madison, WI 53703 or by calling 800-488-4940. Web site: www.taichihealth.com.

Guided Imagery

Think of guided imagery as a daydream with a tour guide. By diverting your attention from stress, guided imagery takes your mind on a mini-vacation. Use your imagination to transport yourself to a more peaceful place. It's up to you to choose where. For some people the most relaxing place is the seashore; for others it's the mountains. Pick your mind's ideal vacation spot, and go there.

Massage

Massage therapy is considered by many to be an excellent way of easing the pain and stiffness associated with arthritis. It can help stretch tight muscles, improve flexibility, and ease pain and stress. Evidence from scientific studies has shown that massage can decrease stress hormones and depression, ease muscle pain and spasms, increase the body's production of natural, pain-killing endorphins, and improve sleep and immune function.

Although there are many different types of massage, most include a combination of strokes, friction and pressure that are used to help relax the muscles. Some types, such as Swedish massage, emphasize the physical by pressing, rubbing and manipulating muscles and joints to improve function. Asian techniques emphasize balancing the flow of vital energy in your body. There are even some techniques – such as reiki and therapeutic touch – that focus on energy for spiritual healing, and practitioners don't physically touch you at all.

What can you expect from your massage? Your session most likely will be given on a padded table or a mat on the floor in a warm, quiet room. It may be softly lit, with quiet music, or it may be more like a typical doctor's office. The therapist should talk to you about any special health conditions or sensitivities, such as actively painful or weak joints, and discuss your goals for the session. You don't have to remove all of your clothes; often, the therapist will cover you with a large sheet and will uncover only the part of your body that is being massaged.

Prayer and Spirituality

A common belief is that prayer and spirituality aid our ability to deal with pain and suffering, comfort us in times of illness and depression, and perhaps aid the healing process. According to behavioral medicine research studies, spiritual activities can have powerful, beneficial effects on our health.

Of course, it is difficult to measure how prayer and faith affect a person's health. One method scientists have used is to observe people who regularly attend religious services, compared with others who refrain. Such studies suggest that people who engage in worship tend to live longer, take better care of their health and recover more quickly from illnesses and depression. Skeptics counter by saying that such studies reveal the benefits of emotional support and community, not religion.

Theories about the possible benefits of prayer suggest that it relieves stress much like meditation does. Praying may calm a person's mind and body.

Whether supported by scientific fact or not, people have found comfort in prayer and other spiritual practices since human history's beginning. Attending worship services or other spiritual activities may be good for you and your arthritis, and it can't hurt you – unless you use it as a substitute for medication or your doctor's prescribed treatment program.

Chapter 14

Emotional Challenges: Handling Grief and Depression

A chronic illness like osteoarthritis can change your life in ways you may never consider until you face them. You may never have thought that some simple tasks like walking down a flight of stairs could become difficult and even painful. Many times after the initial diagnosis, when you become faced with these concerns, grief can set in.

What Is Grief?

In the face of chronic illness such as osteoarthritis, feelings of sadness, frustration, anger and disappointment are normal. Grief is a natural response to loss. We usually think of these feelings in connection with the death of a loved one, but chronic illnesses can involve losses too. For people with osteoarthritis, the losses can be physical, social and personal. Acknowledging these losses is a natural part of the healing process that helps you come to terms with the changes osteoarthritis can bring.

Allowing yourself to grieve can help you to accept losses sooner. And with acceptance, you can begin to move forward again.

Getting Through Grief

Although feelings of grief are a normal response to loss, dealing effectively with these feelings can keep you from becoming overwhelmed by them. Here are some tips to help you cope:

- **Give yourself permission.** Allow yourself to feel sad, angry and upset. Ignoring your feelings and pushing them aside isn't helpful. As long as you don't dwell on them for too long, experiencing these feelings can help you get through them so that you can move on.
- **Examine what triggers these feelings.** Try to figure out which events, situations or fears precede or stir up your feelings of sadness and grief. If certain anniversary

dates, holidays or times of year tend to make you especially sad, plan special activities during those times. Reduce situations that cause you anxiety until you feel better prepared to handle them.

- **Express your feelings, then let go.** Keeping your feelings inside and pushing them down can lead to denial, which can grow into bitterness. Instead, let your feelings out in healthy ways, such as crying, writing in a journal, talking with a friend or punching pillows. Once you let the feelings out, don't continue thinking about them, but release them.
- **Find meaning in your experiences.** Consider what you've learned from your experience and the positive ways osteoarthritis has affected your life. Find the personal gains you've made from taking on this challenge. These may include new priorities, new friends, a better understanding of yourself, strengthened relationships or increased spirituality.
- **Get help if you need it.** Sometimes the practices above are enough to help you deal with grief. But if you're affected more deeply – if you have trouble continuing daily activities, you're feeling hope-

Depression Risk Factors

People are at higher risk for depression at certain times or under certain conditions. You may be at greater risk if:

- You've had a previous episode of depression
- Your previous depressive episode occurred before age 40
- You have a medical condition
- You've just given birth
- You have little or no social support
- You've recently experienced a stressful life event (positive or negative)
- You abuse alcohol or drugs
- You have a family history of depression-related disorders
- You experienced only partial relief from a previous episode of depression.

(Adapted from *Arthritis Today* Magazine)

less, or you're considering harming yourself – seek professional help right away.

What is Depression?

Feelings of grief, sadness and anger are normal responses to loss and to the changes a chronic illness can bring to your life. Although these emotions are normal, if they aren't dealt with properly, they can lead to depression.

Depression has become a popular term to describe a variety of emotional situations and often is used incorrectly to refer to brief feelings of sadness or disappointment. A true depressive disorder, however, is more than that: It profoundly affects how you view yourself and the world.

In fact, depression refers to a broad spectrum of what are known as mood disorders. These include dysthymia, a type of chronic depression in which you experience depressive feelings more days than not over the course of two years or more. The symptoms tend to be mild but persistent. Major depression tends to occur in episodes of more severe symptoms that last for at least two weeks.

It can be difficult to tell that you are depressed when you are experiencing it. The symptoms can start gradually so that you may not realize right away the changes in your outlook. Some medical conditions and medications can induce symptoms similar to depression.

The risk factors on page 158 and self-test on page 160 can help you determine if you may be experiencing depression. If you think you may be depressed, talk with your doctor.

You don't have to continue living with depression. Most depression is treatable with counseling, medications or a combination of the two.

Help for Emotional Challenges

There are several steps you can take to successfully address the emotional challenges of osteoarthritis. The following techniques offer ways you can work through all of the feelings you may experience as a result of a chronic illness like osteoarthritis. These techniques can help you find the strength and support that will allow you to take control and manage these challenges. One technique may work better for you, or for certain situations, so try them all to see which ones you find most effective.

Support Groups

Support groups offer you the chance to share your experiences with others who

Depression Check

It is normal to experience one or more of the following depression symptoms from time to time. But if you've been experiencing a number of these symptoms for weeks or years, you may have a depressive disorder that you should consult your doctor about.

Group 1:

Are you experiencing at least one of the following nearly every day:

- Apathy or loss of interest in things you used to enjoy, including sex
- Sadness, blues or irritability

Group 2:

Are you experiencing any of the following:

- Feeling slowed down or restless
- Feeling worthless or guilty
- Changes in appetite or weight (loss or gain)
- Thoughts of death or suicide
- Problems concentrating, thinking, remembering, or making decisions
- Trouble falling asleep or sleeping too much
- Loss of energy, feeling tired all the time

Group 3:

Are you experiencing any of the following symptoms? These symptoms aren't used to diagnose depression, but they often occur with it.

- Headaches
- Other aches and pains
- Digestive problems
- Sexual problems
- Feeling pessimistic or hopeless
- Feeling anxious or worried
- Low self-esteem

Results:

If you have several of these symptoms, particularly if they last for more than a few days, talk to your doctor. If you are experiencing depression, he or she may be able to recommend an appropriate treatment.

are dealing with the challenges of osteoarthritis. You can take strength and advice from the experiences of others, and gain perspective and solutions for your own problems. Although friends and family certainly offer support, sometimes it can help to have the understanding of others who are facing the same situations. The groups offer support, encouragement, and the chance to see how other people like you are coping with the day-to-day experiences of osteoarthritis.

You can find out about support groups that meet in your area through local hospitals, community centers, senior centers and organizations such as the Arthritis Foundation. You can even join online support groups from the comfort of your own home.

Keeping a Journal

Pouring your thoughts and feelings onto the pages of a journal can be a good way to deal with your emotions. The simple act of writing things down can be a healing experience. It allows you to vent your frustrations privately – without the fear that others may judge you. It also gives

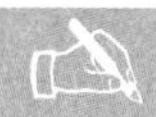

Personally Speaking STORIES FROM REAL PEOPLE

"I have osteoarthritis in my shoulders, knees and hands. But I choose to deal with it – rather than having more surgeries.

THE BENEFITS OF A HEALTH BLITZ

– JAN THORNTON, GLENDALE, CA

"Living with osteoarthritis is a daily challenge to be positive, disciplined, and physically and mentally active. About one year ago, I decided to do a health blitz of swimming and/or walking an hour every morning, taking daily doses of glucosamine and chondroitin, and drinking fresh vegetable and fruit juices. I stopped taking pain killers because they were too hard on my stomach. After this daily regimen, I feel light-years better than before this blitz.

"This undoubtedly will not work for every person. I know it's tempting to be inactive when you first wake up and let the creakiness take over. But it's one of those 'think later – not now' things: you feel so much better when you get up, get moving and get out. In the long run, it pays off."

you the chance to see patterns in your feelings or to see solutions after you've expressed the emotion.

JOURNALING TIPS

- Don't worry about misspellings or the quality of your writing. No one else has to see your journal.
- Consider dating your entries so you can see patterns and progress.
- Don't feel obligated to write every day. Write when you feel you have something to say or to get off your chest. Remember to take time to evaluate your feelings about positive experiences as well as frustrations.

The Arthritis Foundation publishes a ready-made journal called *Toward Healthy Living* that includes inspirational quotes and a scale for monitoring your mood and pain. To order, call 800-283-7800 or visit www.arthritis.org.

Professional Help

A psychiatrist or psychologist can treat disorders like depression. Even if you aren't clinically depressed, a therapist can help you sort through your emotions and find effective ways to deal with them. Therapists also can help you develop better communication skills and strengthen relationships that may be affected by the changes that accompany osteoarthritis.

To find a qualified therapist, begin by asking your doctor for several recommendations. Then ask your insurance company which therapists and services are covered.

Check references and make sure the therapist is licensed. Qualified therapists may be social workers (MSW); psychologists (PhD); psychiatrists (MD); or marriage, family and child counselors (MFCC). Interview potential therapists by phone about their qualifications, approach and areas of expertise. It may be helpful to find someone who has experience in working with people who have chronic illnesses. Make sure you feel comfortable with the therapist, and that his or her approach fits with your expectations and goals for therapy. Most therapists are willing to meet for an initial session so you can make that assessment together.

Chapter 15

Good Living:
Communicating With Family and Friends

Communication is a vital part of any relationship. It is an essential way to show your care and affection for another person, as well as to solve problems and overcome frustration. Because osteoarthritis brings challenges and changes, communication between you and your family and friends is particularly important. You'll need to help them understand the pain and movement limitations that you may experience. You may need to rely on family members or friends for more help with everyday tasks. Open communication can make these transitions in your life go more smoothly, help you feel better about them, and strengthen your relationships with people you care about.

Develop Communication Skills

Good communication practices aren't always easy to follow, especially in difficult or emotional situations. Here are some steps that may help you get through tough discussions:

- **Use "I" messages.** These are factual statements about how you feel that avoid blaming or attacking the other person, but still allow you to be heard. For example, say, "I get frustrated when I'm late," instead of, "You're never ready on time."
- **Remember to express positive feelings.** Don't just think about communicating when there's a problem, communicate affection and appreciation as well.
- **Listen.** Communication isn't only about getting your point across, but also about hearing the other person's side.
- **Don't manipulate.** When you express your thoughts in a way that makes the other person feel guilty or angry, communication will get worse.
- **Look and sound interested.** Make eye contact with the other person and encour-

age him or her during discussions. Nod your head, and even rephrase their words in a different way to make sure you're understanding what the other person means.

Getting the Information You Need

You can't communicate effectively if you don't have all of the information you need. Here are some tips for getting someone to tell you more.

- Ask for more details. It is okay to let the other person know you don't understand what they've told you. Clarify the point with questions like "What do you mean?" or "Can you say that another way?"
- Clarify meaning. Sometimes there are differences between what a person says and what he or she means. Paraphrasing can help you make sure you're getting the message. In your own words, repeat what you believe the other person has said. Avoid an accusatory tone by using phrases such as "Are you saying ..." or "Do you mean ..."
- Be specific. To avoid vague answers, ask specific questions. Instead of asking, "How do you feel?" try, "Are you feeling frustrated?"

Dealing With Anger

Osteoarthritis can stir up anger because of the frustration and uncertainty that accompany chronic illness. The pain and limitations of osteoarthritis are not something you asked for, and your situation can leave you wondering "Why me?"

When you're facing life with arthritis day to day, you can sometimes feel angry at the world, angry at those who are healthy, and angry at the people who try to help you. You may direct your anger toward others or toward yourself.

Many times you may direct your anger toward the friends and family members who are closest to you, especially when you feel that they don't understand your situation or when they don't meet your expectations. For example, if a friend offers you help, you may feel angry because she doesn't see that you can still handle something on your own. Or you might even get angry if she didn't offer to help you, because she wasn't being sensitive enough to realize you needed help.

Although anger is a common response to loss, it can drive away friends and loved ones. Constant angry behavior works against creating and maintaining relationships. Being angry all the time can even make your osteoarthritis pain worse.

Fortunately, there are healthy ways to express your anger. You can even harness the energy and strong feelings that anger brings and use them as a force to help you achieve change.

Because every individual is different, there is no single correct way to deal with anger. There are healthy and unhealthy ways to handle it, however, and certain approaches may be better for certain occasions. Here's a run-down:

Repression. With this approach, you push the unwanted feeling down into your subconscious. If you deny it, you don't have to deal with it, right? But the feeling is still there, and if you don't deal with it, it can fester and grow into bitterness.

Suppression. This method involves a conscious attempt to hold back your feelings of anger. Hold back too long, and the suppressed anger can lead to a blowup.

At other times, suppression can be a useful, healthy tool. You can hold back the anger for a short time until you can deal with it appropriately. For the moment, take a deep breath, count to 10 and hold your tongue.

Expression. This way of handling your anger is sometimes healthy and sometimes unhealthy. Unhealthy expression includes passive/aggressive behavior such as complaining under your breath, being stubborn, or using silence to control other people.

Healthy expression, however, is a constructive way to use anger, without trying to assert superiority over someone or gain special treatment because of your illness. You choose a purposeful goal for your anger rather than reacting unconsciously and aggressively. You are sensitive to the other person's responsiveness by choosing a time when he or she is most open to what you have to say. It can help to

Anger Check

Use the following questions to evaluate how you express your anger:

- What are your sources of anger?
- What other emotions may be coming out as anger – guilt, fear, hurt?
- Who are the innocent people you turn your anger against?
- What are the ways you use to process your feelings of anger? Are they healthy or unhealthy ways?

Adapted from *Celebrate Life: New Attitudes for Living with Chronic Illness* by Kathleen Lewis. To order, call 800-283-7800 or order online at www.arthritis.org.

express your anger to someone completely uninvolved in the situation and outside of your immediate circle so that you get it out and move on.

Release. Find creative ways to blow off steam, release tension and get through your anger. Exercise is a great outlet, especially because you need to do it any-

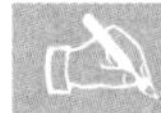

Personally Speaking STORIES FROM REAL PEOPLE

FRIENDS AND THE ARTHRITIS FOUNDATION

– ELINOR ROBIN SLAVITSKY, FORT LEE, NJ

"I have osteoarthritis in the lumbar and thoracic spine, in both hands, and most recently, in my left shoulder. I take my medication daily, hoping that one day there will be a cure for this disease so all victims will be free of pains and aches. I have my back brace, cane and hand splints to wear when I am in extreme pain.

"I developed osteoarthritis in 1994, and never knew I had it until I had a physical exam with my primary care doctor, who suggested an orthopaedic doctor examine me. I went through X-rays, MRIs and all sorts of medications, such as *Daypro*, *Celebrex* and now *Relafen*.

"After that, I wanted to become a member of an organization that helps others with this disease, which is why I became a member of the Arthritis Foundation. I continuously pledged my fees. But then it became apparent to me: 'Why don't I name the Foundation in my will?' I called, and the Foundation gave me what I needed about Planned Giving and naming the Arthritis Foundation in my will.

"After pledging yearly, I was honored as a Lifetime Member of the Foundation. I received a magnificent plaque with my name on it, two gold pins, and a beautiful, personalized letter from the president and CEO of the Foundation.

"Having this disease is not fun or enjoyable. I have pain daily so I exercise, walk, swim and eat a proper diet. I have the support of friends and, most important, of Howard, my husband, who has been with me through good, bad, happy and sad times. I pray to God each and every day that arthritis and all its forms will be cured and gone forever."

way and you can let out your frustrations at the same time. Choose a private place and scream as loud as you can. Punch a pile of pillows or write your feelings in your journal.

Asking for Help

Learning that you cannot do everything yourself and asking others to pitch in are keys to being a successful self-manager. You can learn to delegate the tasks of managing your activities.

At first, it may be awkward to ask for help. Because the effects of osteoarthritis are not always visible to others, you may fear that co-workers and acquaintances will think you are lazy. That may bother you, especially if you've always prided yourself on being a high achiever.

The following suggestions can ease the process of asking for help from others.

- **Ask for specific help.** If you ask someone to take you to the supermarket for one hour every other Friday afternoon, you are letting them know precisely the help you need. Also, you show them that you realize their time is valuable.
- **Develop a "pool" of helpers.** Keep the burden from falling on any one relative or friend by spreading the load of tasks. Make a list of friends and family and how much help each person can provide.
- **Consider bartering or trading services with others.** If you feel uncomfortable asking for help, perhaps you can reciprocate. For instance, you can offer to take your friend's children to the playground one afternoon a week in exchange for helping you with your weekly grocery shopping.

Responding to "How Are You?"

This common question has become something we all take for granted in everyday social situations. It becomes a bit more tricky, however, when you have osteoarthritis and the automatic response of "Fine" doesn't come quite so easily.

How you really feel can change, depending on how much your symptoms are affecting you at different points in the day. Maybe you're unsure whether the person really wants to know how you are doing or whether they're just being polite. Answering does become easier as you become more comfortable with yourself and with osteoarthritis. Here are a few tips to get you started:

- Sometimes it may be best to downplay your condition, for instance at work or when you are meeting someone new.
- At other times, you need to be more honest about exactly how you are feeling –

with your doctor, for example, or with close, understanding family and friends.

- It may be best to keep it short with responses like "I'm getting by" or "I'm hanging in there."
- Make a list of other responses you feel comfortable with so that you're ready when someone asks.

Getting Past Codependency

In a codependent relationship, each partner plays a role of victim or rescuer. In this situation, one partner is always ready to rush in and rescue the other at the hint of a problem. This encourages the ill partner to assume the victim role.

For the rescuer, the thought of the victim not needing their help may be so threatening that deep down he or she may not wish for the victim to get better. And the caretaker may try to presume what the victim wants, only to be met with hostility and resentment. In the end, both partners become victims.

This is an easy trap to fall into, especially when you have a chronic illness like osteoarthritis. To balance a tendency toward codependency, try using "I" statements to set your boundaries. For example, you may say "I can dress myself" and "I need help with the chores today," instead of "You don't have to help me" and "You never do anything around here." These "You" statements place blame rather than state the case.

Talking With Your Partner About Sexuality

A chronic illness like osteoarthritis can affect your sexuality in several ways. Painful joints may make you reluctant to consider sexual intimacy because it could add to your pain. Reduced range of motion can make sex more difficult. And arthritis can affect your feelings of attractiveness and desire so that you may feel less interested in sex.

But if you don't communicate these feelings to your partner, he or she could misinterpret your withdrawal from sexual activity as rejection, which in turn could harm your relationship.

Talk with your partner about how osteoarthritis affects your feelings about sexual intimacy. Discuss your needs and desires, and help your partner understand what feels good and what doesn't.

Encourage your partner to express his or her feelings as well. He or she may be concerned that sex could be painful for you, and may feel anxious about intimacy.

Avoiding sex could cause tension in your relationship, so don't let feelings and concerns go unsaid.

Rekindling the Romance

If osteoarthritis has affected your sexual relationship with your partner, consider the following suggestions to make sex more comfortable and to rekindle feelings of intimacy.

- **Be prepared.** With osteoarthritis, you may need to plan ahead for sexual intimacy. Get pain under control by taking your medication or using heat or cold treatments. Try doing some mild stretching beforehand to ease stiff joints.
- **Be creative – and gentle.** Sex can be a tender, healing experience. And it doesn't always have to include intercourse. Sometimes a little romance and a gentle massage when you're in pain can foster emotional and physical closeness.
- **Talk to your doctor**. Other factors such as medications or feelings of depression can affect interest in sex. Your doctor can help assess the problem and find a solution, like treating the depression or adjusting your medication.
- **Find ways to feel good in your body.** The physical effects of arthritis can affect your feelings of attractiveness. Think of

Talk to Your Partner

Talking with your partner about sexual intimacy can help you both feel better and improve your relationship. Here are some questions to think about and discuss with your partner:

- Has osteoarthritis altered your sexual relationship or your feelings about your sexuality?
- What has changed, if anything?
- What has stayed the same?
- Are any sexual activities less pleasant than they used to be?
- Are any more enjoyable?
- Does sexual intimacy cause any problems for you or your partner?
- Where do you enjoy being touched and where do you not?
- Are there new things you would like to try?

Adapted from the Arthritis Foundation's *Systemic Lupus Erythematosus Self-Help Course*, 1994

ways to feel good about yourself. Appeal to your senses by lighting candles and using satin or flannel sheets. Wear clothes that make you look and feel good. Do exercise that allows you to enjoy moving your body.

- **Be romantic and reassuring.** Try making romantic gestures that let your partner know how much you love and care about him or her. Let each other know what makes you feel loved, and try to do those things.

For additional information and advice on dealing with sexuality, intimacy and arthritis, request a free copy of the *Arthritis Foundation's Guide to Intimacy*, reprinted from *Arthritis Today* magazine. Call 800-568-4045 or visit www.arthritis.org to request your copy.

A Final Word

Now that you've finished this book, you have the tools to live better with osteoarthritis. As a final note, let's review the key steps to good living with osteoarthritis and how they can help you.

- **Understand osteoarthritis.** Knowledge is power, so learn as much as you can about how osteoarthritis affects your body and how it can be treated. Keep yourself informed about the latest research and treatments for osteoarthritis by reading and researching on your own.
- **Become a self-manager.** Become involved in your own health care. Do whatever you can to control the aspects of the disease that you can influence. Follow your prescribed treatment plan, and take part in monitoring your progress.
- **Adopt a wellness lifestyle.** Take steps to live a healthy life in general. Wellness practices include taking care of your body and your mind, and having a positive outlook toward life. Incorporating wellness practices into your daily life can help you feel better, too.
- **Exercise.** Exercise is one of the most effective ways to reduce pain and protect your joints because it strengthen the muscles around them. Develop an exercise program you can enjoy and maintain.
- **Maintain a healthy weight.** Along with exercising, keeping your weight down is one of the best things you can do for your joints. If you're overweight, take steps to lose weight by modifying your diet and stepping up your exercise program to prevent further stress and damage to your joints.
- **Manage pain.** This book has offered you a number of strategies for managing the pain of osteoarthritis. Some may work better than others for you or may be better for certain situations. Experiment with the strategies and create a pain-management plan that works for you. Then use those techniques to keep your pain at bay.
- **Handle stress and emotional challenges.** Chronic illness can bring a number of changes to your life that can affect you emotionally. Learn to take control of these emotional challenges by managing stress effectively. Seek help if the emotional aspect of chronic illness becomes more serious than you can handle alone.

Glossary

acupressure: Eastern medicine technique in which pressure is applied to specific sites along energy pathways called meridians.

acupuncture: Eastern medicine technique in which needles are used to puncture the body at specific sites along energy pathways called meridians.

acute illness: Disease that can be severe but of short duration, unlike chronic illness.

acute pain: See pain.

aerobic: An activity designed to increase oxygen consumption, such as aerobic exercise or aerobic breathing.

alternative therapy: Any practice or substance outside the realm of conventional medicine.

American College of Rheumatology (ACR): An organization that provides a professional, educational, and research forum for rheumatologists across the country. Among its functions: helping determine what symptoms and signs define rheumatic disease diagnoses and what the treatments are for those diagnoses.

analgesic: Drugs used to help relieve pain.

anesthesia: Chemicals that induce a partial or complete loss of sensation. Used to perform surgery and other medical procedures.

anesthesiologist: A physician specializing in the administration of anesthesia.

arthritis: From the Greek word "arth" meaning "joint," and the suffix "itis" meaning "inflammation." A condition involving pain and/or damage in or around the joints, stemming from any cause such as infection, trauma or inflammation.

arthrodesis: A surgical procedure fusing two bones.

arthroplasty: A surgical procedure that replaces a joint with an artificial one.

arthroscopic surgery: A type of surgery using an instrument called an arthroscope, which consists of a thin tube with a light at one end. The arthroscope is inserted into the body through a small incision and connected to a closed-circuit television.

aspiration: The removal of a substance by suction. Technique used to remove fluid from an inflamed joint, both to relieve pressure and to examine the fluid.

ASU: A mixture of avocado and soybean oils taken as a dietary supplement to ease osteoarthritis pain.

biomedical model: Traditional model of medical care, based on the principle of identifying a single cause and cure for each disease.

biopsychosocial model: More recent model of medical care than the traditional one, in which a patient's self-management plays a part in the treatment of chronic disease.According to this model, biological, psychological and socioeconomic factors are considered influential to the disease's outcome.

body mechanics: The structures and methods with which your body moves and performs physical tasks.

boron: A trace mineral that helps the body use nutrients such as calcium and magnesium. Taken as a supplement, it may ease osteoarthritis symptoms.

boswellia: Also known as frankincense and derived from an Asian tree. Combined with other herbs, it may ease osteoarthritis symptoms.

bunion: Inflammation, enlargement and malalignment of the joint of the toe.

bursa: A small sac located between a tendon and a bone. The bursae (plural for bursa) reduce friction and provide lubrication. See also bursitis.

bursitis: Inflammation of a bursa (see bursa) that can occur when the joint has been overused or when the joint has become deformed by arthritis. Bursitis makes it painful to move or put pressure on the affected joint.

capsaicin: A chemical contained in some hot peppers. Capsaicin gives these peppers their burn and has painkilling properties. It is available in nonprescription creams that can be rubbed on the skin over a joint to relieve pain.

cardiovascular: Related to the heart and blood vessels.

cartilage: A firm, smooth, rubbery substance that provides a gliding surface for joint motion, and prevents bone-on-bone contact.

chiropodist: A doctor with particular training in the care of the feet. Also called podiatrist.

chiropractic: Practice of healing based on spinal manipulation and the belief that illness stems from malalignment of the spinal cord.

chiropractor: Also known as a doctor of chiropractic, a health professional certified in chiropractic. Not licensed to perform surgery or prescribe drugs.

chondroitin sulfate: Dietary supplement derived from cattle trachea, purported to help stop joint degeneration, improve function and ease pain. Part of a naturally occurring protein in human cartilage that gives it elasticity.

chronic illness: Disease that is of a long duration, such as osteoarthritis.

chronic pain: Pain that is constant or persists over a long period, perhaps for life. See pain.

collagen: A protein that is the primary component of cartilage. See cartilage.

complementary therapy: Any practice or substance used in conjunction with traditional treatment.

cool-down exercises: A series of physical activities that allow your heart and respiration rates to normalize after exercise.

corticosteroids: A group of hormones including cortisol produced by the adrenal glands. They can be synthetically produced (i.e., made in a laboratory) and have powerful anti-inflammatory effects. Although they are sometimes called corticosteroids or steroids, they are not the same as the dangerous performance-enhancing drugs that some athletes use to promote strength and endurance.

cortisone: A hormone produced by the cortex of the adrenal gland. Cortisone has potent anti-inflammatory effects but also can have side effects. See also corticosteroids.

counterirritants: Topical analgesics that contain substances such as wintergreen oil, camphor or eucalyptus oil, which stimulate nerve endings and distract the brain from joint pain.

COX-2 drugs: Also known as COX-2 inhibitors, drugs that inhibit inflammation without the gastrointestinal side effects of traditional NSAIDs. Includes celecoxib.

deconditioning: Loss of muscle mass and strength because of inactivity. See also reconditioning.

deep breathing: Drawing air into the lungs, filling them as much as possible, and then exhaling slowly. Performing this type of rhythmic breathing for a few minutes increases the amount of oxygen reaching your brain and produces relaxation and readiness for mental tasks.

depression: A state of mind characterized by gloominess, dejection or sadness.

depression, clinical: A recognized mental illness in which the feelings of depression are severe, prolonged and hamper your ability to function normally.

depression, major: A term for a chronic clinical depression involving severe, persistent symptoms.

disease: Sickness. Some physicians use this term only for conditions that involve a structural or functional change in tissues or organs.

disorder: An ailment; an abnormal health condition.

double-jointedness: Also known as joint laxity, this is an inherited trait that allows the joints to bend farther than usual.

dysthmia: A type of chronic depression with mild, but persistent symptoms.

endorphins: Natural painkillers produced by the nervous system with qualities similar to opiate drugs. Endorphins are released during exercise and laughter.

endurance exercises: Exercises such as swimming, walking and cycling that use the large muscles of the body and are dependent on increasing the amount of oxygen that reaches the muscles. These strengthen muscles and increase and maintain physical fitness.

ergonomics: The study of human capabilities and limitations in relation to the work system, machine or task, as well as the study of the physical, psychological and social environment of the worker. Also known as "human engineering."

erythrocyte sedimentation rate: A test measuring how fast red blood cells (erythrocytes) fall to the bottom of a test tube, indicating level of inflammation. Often called *ESR* or *sed rate.*

fatigue: A general worn-down feeling and lack of energy. Fatigue can be caused by excessive physical, mental or emotional exertion, by lack of sleep, and by inflammation or disease.

fibromyalgia: A noninfectious rheumatic condition affecting the body's soft tissue. Characterized by muscle pain, fatigue and nonrestorative sleep, fibromyalgia produces no abnormal X-ray or laboratory findings. It is often associated with headaches and irritable bowel syndrome.

flare: A term used to describe times when the disease or condition is at its worst.

flexibility exercises: Muscle stretches and other activities designed to maintain flexibility and to prevent stiffness or shortening of ligaments and tendons.

Food Labeling Act: 1994 legal decree of the U.S. government mandating the type of information that must be given on food labels regarding nutritional content. This act ensures that consumers will have easy-to-read fat, protein, fiber, carbohydrate and calorie content information, and more.

gate control theory: A theory of how pain signals travel to the brain. According to this theory, pain signals must pass a "pain gate" that can be opened or closed by various positive (e.g., feelings of happiness) or negative (e.g., feelings of sadness) factors.

ginger: Root that, when taken in the form of tea or supplement capsules, may relieve pain and inflammation.

glucosamine: An amino sugar that appears to play a role in cartilage formation and repair. Taken as a dietary supplement derived from crab, lobster and shrimp shells, it may relieve pain.

gout: Disease that occurs due to an excess of uric acid in the blood, causing crystals to deposit in the joint, leading to pain and inflammation.

grief: Feelings of loss; acute sorrow.

guided imagery: A method of managing pain and stress. The voice of a guide, an audiotape or videotape, or your own internal voice focuses your attention on a series of images that lead your mind away from the stress or pain.

hormones: Concentrated chemical substances produced in the glands or organs that have specific – and usually multiple – regulatory effects on the body.

hyaluronan: A substance in the synovial fluid of the joint, giving it viscosity, or thickness, and helping the joint absorb shock. See viscosupplementation.

illness: Poor health; sickness.

inflammation: A response to injury or infection that involves a sequence of biochemical reactions. Inflammation can be generalized, causing fatigue, fever, and pain or tenderness all over the body. It can be localized, for example, in joints, where it causes swelling and pain.

internist: A physician who specializes in internal medicine, sometimes called a primary-care physician.

isometric exercises: Exercises that build the muscles around joints by tightening the muscles without moving the joints.

isotonic exercises: Exercises that strengthen muscles by moving the joints.

joint: The place or part where one bone connects to another.

joint aspiration: Also known as arthrocentesis, a laboratory test in which fluid is drained from the joint and examined for crystals or joint deterioration. See aspiration.

joint count: An examination done by a doctor to determine the number of joints that are affected by arthritis.

joint malalignment: When joints are not aligned properly, due to joint damage.

joint replacement surgery: Also known as arthroplasty, a surgical procedure involving the reconstruction or replacement (with a man-made component) of a joint.

ligament: Flexible band of fibrous tissue

that connects bones to one another.

malalignment, joint: When joints are not aligned properly, due to joint damage.

massage: A technique of applying pressure, friction or vibration to the muscles, by hand or using a massage appliance, to stimulate circulation and produce relaxation and pain relief.

massage therapist: One who has completed a program of study and is licensed to perform massage.

meditation: A sustained period of deep inward thought, reflection and openness to inspiration.

meridians: Energy pathways used in Eastern medicine, which have no Western medicine counterparts.

morbidity rate: The frequency or proportion of people with a particular diagnosis or disability in a given population.

MRI: Magnetic Resonance Imaging test, a scan used as a diagnostic aid.

muscle: Tissue that moves organs or parts of the body.

myalgia: Pain of the muscles.

NSAID (nonsteroidal anti-inflammatory drug): A type of drug that does not contain steroids but is used to relieve pain and reduce inflammation.

nurse: A person who has received education and training in health care, particularly patient care. Many nurses have earned a registered nurse degree, noted by RN in their title.

nurse practitioner: A registered nurse with advanced training emphasizing primary care.

occupational therapist: A health professional who teaches patients to reduce strain on joints while doing everyday activities.

orthopaedic surgeon: A surgeon who specializes in diseases of the bone.

orthopaedist: A physician who specializes in diseases of the bone.

orthotic devices: Splints and braces that support and protect joints.

osteoarthritis: A disease causing cartilage breakdown in certain joints (spine, hands, hips, knees), resulting in pain and deformity.

osteophytes: Bony spurs that develop on the ends of bones. Can occur in osteoarthritis as a result of cartilage breakdown.

osteoporosis: A disease that causes bones to lose their mass and break easily.

osteotomy: A surgical procedure involving the cutting of bone, usually performed in cases of severe joint malalignment.

pain: A sensation or perception of hurting, ranging from discomfort to agony, which occurs in response to injury, disease or functional disorder. Pain is your body's alarm system, signaling that something is wrong. Acute pain is temporary, related to nerve endings stimulated by tissue damage, and improves with healing. Chronic pain may be mild to severe, but persists due to tissue damage or pain impulses that keep the pain gate open.

pharmacist: A professional licensed to prepare and dispense drugs.

physiatrist: A physician who continues training after medical school and specializes in the field of physical medicine and rehabilitation.

physical therapist: A person who has professional training and is licensed in the practice of physical therapy.

physical therapy: Methods and techniques of rehabilitation to restore function and prevent disability following injury or disease. Methods may include applications of heat and cold, assistive devices, massage, and an individually tailored program of exercises.

physician: A person who has successfully completed medical school and is licensed to practice medicine. Also known as a doctor.

physician, family: See physician, primary-care.

physician, general practitioner: See physician, primary-care.

physician, osteopathic: Doctors, also known as osteopaths, who base diagnosis and treatment on a philosophy that many illnesses are connected to disorders in the musculoskeletal system. Osteopaths have the same level of training as medical doctors and may be primary care physicians or specialists, such as rheumatologists.

physician, primary-care: Physician to whom a family or individual goes when ill or for a periodic health check. For the patient with multiple health concerns, this physician assumes medical coordination of care with other physicians.

physician's assistant: A person trained, certified and licensed to assist physicians by recording medical history and performing a physical examination, diagnosis and treatment of commonly encountered medical problems under the supervision of a licensed physician.

placebo effect: The phenomenon in which a person receiving an inactive drug or therapy experiences a reduction in symptoms.

podiatrist: A health professional who specializes in care of the foot. Formerly called a chiropodist.

polyarthritis: Arthritis affecting many joints.

polymyalgia rheumatica: Disease causing joint and muscle pain, morning stiffness and a feeling of malaise. Marked by a high erythrocyte sedimentation rate and occasionally by fever.

psychiatrist: A physician who trains after medical school in the study, treatment and prevention of mental disorders. A psychiatrist may provide counseling and prescribe medicines and other therapies.

psychologist: A trained professional, usually not a medical doctor, who specializes in the mind and mental processes, especially in relation to human and animal behavior. A psychologist may measure mental abilities and provide counseling.

psychosomatic: Pertaining to the link between the mind (psyche) and the body (soma).

range of motion (ROM): The distance and angles at which your joints can be moved, extended and rotated in various directions.

reconditioning: Restoring or improving muscle tone and strength with appropriate and balanced exercise, nutrition and rest. See also deconditioning.

rehabilitation counselor: A person who guides physical and mental rehabilitation.

relaxation: A state of release from mental or physical stress or tension.

repression: Denying feelings (such as anger) or pushing them into the subconscious.

resection: Surgical procedure removing all or part of a bone.

resection arthroplasty: A surgical procedure in which resection is done in conjunction with arthroplasty.

revision: A surgical procedure to replace an artificial joint.

rheumatic disease: A general term referring to conditions characterized by pain and stiffness of the joints or muscles. The American College of Rheumatology currently recognizes more than 100 rheumatic diseases. The term often is used interchangeably with *arthritis* (meaning joint inflammation), but not all rheumatic diseases affect the joints or involve inflammation.

rheumatoid arthritis: A chronic, inflammatory autoimmune disease in which the body's protective immune system turns on the body and attacks the joints, causing pain, swelling and deformity.

rheumatologist: A physician who pursues additional training after medical school and specializes in the diagnosis, treatment and prevention of arthritis and other rheumatic disorders.

rheumatologist, pediatric: A rheumatologist who specializes in the diagnosis, treatment, and prevention of arthritis or other rheumatic diseases in children and adolescents.

salicylates: A subcategory of NSAIDs, including aspirin. Also describes topical creams that relieve pain and inflammation.

SAM-e: Supplement purported to relieve pain and possibly ease depression symptoms. Short for S-adenosylmethionine.

self-efficacy: Emotional control in reaction to life events, such as a chronic illness.

self-help: Any course, activity, or action that you do to improve your circumstances or ability to cope with a situation.

self-management: Controlling your disease and its management.

self-talk: The voice you use to talk to yourself, out loud or in thought.

skeletal muscles: The voluntary muscles that are primarily involved in moving parts of the body. "Voluntary" in this sense refers to muscles that move in response to our decisions to walk, bend, grasp and so on, as opposed to muscles such as the heart, which work without our conscious direction.

social worker: A person who has professional training and is licensed to help people capitalize on their own resources and those of social services (for example, home nursing care or vocational rehabilitation).

soft-tissue rheumatism: Pertaining to the many rheumatic conditions affecting the soft (as opposed to the hard or bony) tissues of the body. Fibromyalgia is one type of soft-tissue rheumatism. Others are bursitis, tendinitis and myofascial pain.

steroids: A group name for lipids (fat substances) produced in the body and sharing a particular type of chemical structure. Among these are bile acids, cholesterol, and some hormones. Not the same as anabolic steroids, drugs synthesized from testosterone (the male sex hormone), and used by some athletes to promote strength and endurance.

strain: Injury to a muscle, tendon or ligament by repetitive use, trauma or excessive stretching.

strengthening exercises: Exercises that help maintain or increase muscle strength. See also isometric exercises and isotonic exercises.

stress: The body's physical, mental and chemical reactions to frightening, exciting, dangerous or irritating circumstances.

stressor: Factors that cause stress in your life.

suppression: Holding back feelings, such as anger.

syndrome: A collection of symptoms and/or physical findings that characterize an abnormal condition or illness.

synovectomy: Surgical removal of the synovium, or the lining of the joint.

synovitis: Inflammation of the lining of the joint.

synovium: The lining of the joint.

synovial fluid: The fluid found in the joint.

tai chi: Ancient Chinese practice that involves gentle, fluid movements and meditation to help strengthen muscles, improve balance and relieve stress.

target heart rate: The number of heartbeats per minute that people want to reach during exercise in order to gain maximum benefits. Because the normal heart rate changes as we age, target heart rates are grouped by age.

tendinitis: Inflammation of a tendon.

tendon: A cord of dense, fibrous tissue uniting a muscle to a bone.

TENS: a treatment for pain involving a small device that directs mild electric pulses to nerves in the painful area.

tissue: A collection of similar cells that act together to perform a specific function in the body. The primary tissues are epithelial (skin), connective (ligaments and tendons), bone, muscle and nervous.

uric acid: Substance formed when the body breaks down waste products called *purines*. Uric acid crystals deposited in the joints cause gout.

viscosupplementation: A treatment for knee osteoarthritis involving an injection of a hyaluronic acid product (see viscosupplements) into the joint.

viscosupplements: Products injected to replace the hyaluronic acid missing from knee joints affected by osteoarthritis.

visual analogue scale: A tool used to measure subjective feelings, such as pain, on a scale of 0 to 10 or 0 to 100; used to track disease progress and the effectiveness of pain medications.

warm-up: Gentle movement to warm up the muscles before performing stretches and more strenuous exercise.

yoga: Meaning "union," an ancient Indian practice that involves a series of body postures called *asanas*. Yoga includes exercise, meditation and breathing components to improve posture and balance and help relieve stress on the

INDEX

A

B

C

D

I

J

K

L

M

N

O

S

Resources for Good Living

The Arthritis Foundation, the only national, voluntary health organization that works for the more than 66 million Americans with arthritis or chronic joint symptoms, offers many valuable resources through more than 150 offices nationwide. Your local chapter has information, products, classes and other services to help you take control of your arthritis or related condition. To find the chapter office nearest you, call 800-568-4045 or search the Arthritis Foundation Web site at www.arthritis.org.

Programs and Services

- Physician referral – Most Arthritis Foundation chapters can provide a list of doctors in your area who specialize in the evaluation and treatment of arthritis and arthritis-related diseases.
- Exercise programs – The Arthritis Foundation sponsors, develops and coordinates exercise programs for people with arthritis, featuring specially-trained instructors. They include:

  1) *Walk With Ease* – This course allows participants to develop a walking plan that meets their individual needs, accompanied by the Arthritis Foundation book *Walk With Ease: Your Guide to Walking for Better Health, Improved Fitness and Less Pain*. An audio walking guide is now available to use during your walking routines, with guidelines, upbeat music and inspiring motivation. In addition, a *Walk With Ease* group leader's manual is available to help you start and lead a walking group in your area.
  2) *Arthritis Foundation Exercise Program* – Relieve stiffness and lessen arthritis pain by doing low-impact exercises designed for people with arthritis and taught by trained instructors.
  3) *Arthritis Foundation Aquatic Program* – Join in the fun of a six- to 10-week exercise program in an heated pool led by trained instructors.
  4) *Arthritis Foundation Self-Help Program* – Learn how to take control of your own care in this six-week class for people with arthritis. This program was developed at Stanford University.

Information and Products

Find the latest information about arthritis, including research, medications, government advocacy, programs and services through one of the many information resources offered by the Arthritis Foundation:

- www.arthritis.org – Information about arthritis is available 24 hours a day on the

Internet at the Arthritis Foundation's interactive, comprehensive Web site. Find news about arthritis, ways to get involved, and a variety of useful arthritis products, including books, brochures, videos and more.

• Arthritis Answers – Call toll-free at 800-568-4045 for 24-hour, automated information about arthritis and Arthritis Foundation resources. Trained volunteers and staff are also available at your local Arthritis Foundation chapter to answer questions or refer you to physicians and other resources. Or e-mail questions to help@arthritis.org.

• Books – The Arthritis Foundation publishes a variety of books on arthritis to help you learn to understand and manage your condition, live a healthier life, and cope with the emotional challenges that come with a chronic illness. Order books directly at www.arthritis.org or by calling 800-283-7800. Most Arthritis Foundation books are available at your local bookstore.

• Brochures – The Arthritis Foundation offers brochures containing concise, understandable information on the many arthritis-related diseases and conditions. Topics include surgery, the latest medications, guidance for working with your doctors and self-managing your illness. Single copies are available free of charge at www.arthritis.org or by calling 800-568-4045.

• *Arthritis Today* – This award-winning bimonthly magazine provides the latest information on research, new treatments, trends and tips from experts and readers to help you manage arthritis. A one-year subscription to *Arthritis Today* is included when you become a member of the Arthritis Foundation. Annual membership is $20 and helps fund research to find cures for arthritis. Call 800-283-7800 for information.

• *Kids Get Arthritis Too* – This newsletter focusing on juvenile rheumatic diseases, is published six times a year. Features speak to children and teens with the illness as well as to their parents. Stories examine the latest news in diagnosis, treatment and research of children's rheumatic diseases, as well as helpful ways kids can cope with their illnesses and the challenges they bring. This newsletter is free. To sign up, e-mail kgatmail@arthritis.org or write *Kids Get Arthritis Too*, 1330 West Peachtree Street, NW, Suite 100, Atlanta, GA 30309.